DID YOU KNOW?

- Vitamin E oil can help heal diaper rash
- Ginger tea can make a stomachache feel better
- Garlic can help ward off head lice
- Cayenne pepper can help combat frostbite
- Vitamin C can help reduce inflammation associated with an ear infection
- A sponge bath with eucalyptus oil helps relieve fever
- A pressure point behind the earlobe can help stop hiccups
- Jewelweed not only counteracts the effects of poison ivy, it usually grows right next to it

Give your child these gentle treatments, and many more as you learn about . . .

NATURAL HEALING FOR CHILDREN

NATURAL HEALING

•• F O R ••

CHILDREN

An Essential Handbook for Parents

Winifred Conkling

A LYNN SONBERG BOOK

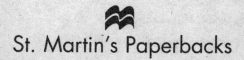

St. Martin's Paperbacks

Published by arrangement with:
Lynn Sonberg Book Associates
260 West 72nd Street, Suite 6-C
New York, NY 10023
212 874-4348

NATURAL HEALING FOR CHILDREN

ISBN: 0-312-96044-1

Printed in the United States of America

St. Martin's Paperbacks edition/January 1997

10 9 8 7 6 5 4 3

IMPORTANT NOTE
TO READERS:

This book is not intended to take the place of medical advice from a trained medical professional. It was written to educate the public concerning conventional and alternative medical treatments for common children's ailments. Parents are advised to consult a pediatrician or other qualified health professional regarding treatment of all of their children's health problems. Neither the publisher, the producer, nor the author take any responsibility for any possible consequences from any treatment, action, or application of medicine or preparation by any person reading or following the information in this book.

For Mandy Prigg Bolgiano,
who always has an open mind and
an open heart

•• Natural Healing for Children ••

•• Introduction ••

As every parent is painfully aware, it's impossible to usher a little one through childhood without experiencing a number of accidents, illnesses, and medical maladies. Face it: Your kid is going to fall and trip and get into accidents (and you'll blame yourself for many of them), in addition to coming down with strange rashes and virtually every infectious disease being passed around at school. And when your child is sick or injured, she's going to come looking for you to make it all better.

In most cases, the common afflictions of childhood prove to be little more than a nuisance, but even the most trivial episode may seem traumatic when it's happening to *your* child. That's why parents need as much medical information as possible when dealing with common childhood illnesses. *Natural Remedies for Children* provides parents with the information they need, including advice on both traditional treatments and natural approaches to healing.

Part 1 of this book provides an overview of natural medicine and outlines the philosophy and practice of four natural approaches to healing: diet and nutrition, herbal medicine, homeopathy, and acupressure. Part 2 is an alphabetical series of entries describing specific childhood ailments and their treatments. Since "an ounce of prevention is worth a pound of cure," each entry also includes practical tips on prevention whenever appropriate.

The information presented in this book is safe and accurate,

1

and most of the medical problems covered in the book can be dealt with at home. However, even the most seemingly mundane conditions demand professional medical care when complications arise. The difficulty, of course, is determining when to seek professional medical care and when to try to get your worries in check. To help parents figure out when to call for help, each entry includes a section that describes warning signs and symptoms that warrant a call or visit to the doctor. If your child is seriously ill or does not respond to the treatments listed here, promptly seek the care of a trained medical professional.

· PART 1 ·

Natural Medicines, Natural Cures

Natural Medicine:
A Different Approach to
Childhood Ailments

We live in an age of medical miracles. Antibiotics cure bacterial infections that killed people in the recent past. Doctors can transplant organs, take three-dimensional pictures of the brain, and even operate on babies with serious health problems before they are born. Despite these impressive advances, there are times when thousand-year-old natural remedies are every bit as effective—or more so—than traditional medical treatments.

When faced with a serious illness or major injury, few Americans would dismiss traditional medical treatment, but many have become disillusioned with the way conventional medicine handles common ailments and everyday aches and pains. And now more than ever, people realize that they don't have to choose between traditional medicine and natural medicine, and instead can embrace both approaches to healing.

Alternative Approaches

Natural medicine is based on one simple truth: The human body has considerable power to heal itself. Wounds heal, rashes disappear, illnesses run their course. Herbalists, homeopaths, acupressurists, and other practitioners of natural medicine attempt to facilitate the healing process by taking into account the whole patient, not just the part that is sick or injured. Practitioners of natural medicine have an interconnected, holistic vision of how the human body works—and of how the body heals itself. Practitioners of conventional medicine, on the other hand, tend to focus on controlling symptoms of disease or injury, using drugs and surgery to deal with specific complaints or conditions.

In recent years, natural medicine has come into its own. Many medical organizations that in the past had spoken out against natural medicine now endorse many of the same recommendations that practitioners of natural medicine have been making for decades. For example, naturopaths have long recommended that people eat high-fiber foods, exercise on a regular basis, reduce stress, and cut back on the intake of refined sugars, fats, and food additives. Now, after decades of debate, many conventional practitioners support these same suggestions.

Likewise, herbal remedies, acupressure, and other natural methods of healing are being taught in mainstream hospital centers and medical schools, places where the techniques were eschewed not long ago. Even the renowned National Institutes of Health opened an Office of Alternative Medicine in 1993, and began funding research on various alternative medical techniques.

Natural medicine is taking its place next to traditional medicine, especially in the treatment of relatively minor conditions. If your child comes down with a serious illness or suffers a major injury, by all means head for the doctor, but to stave off a cold or deal with diarrhea, you might want to try an alternative treatment. No single system of medicine provides all the answers all the time. A cooperative approach to medical care, which includes both traditional treatments and natural remedies, may provide the best care for your child's health.

··2··

Diet and Nutrition: Food, Vitamins, and Nutrition Supplements

Kids don't always eat what they should, even when their parents go to great lengths to provide nutritious meals and healthy snacks. When kids consistently turn up their noses at vegetables and beg for burgers and fries, many parents wonder whether they should supplement their daily bread with a daily vitamin.

In virtually all cases, the answer is yes. A well-balanced diet is a cornerstone to good health for children and adults alike, but multivitamins and nutrition supplements can come in handy when you want to make up for dietary failings, as long as you follow the package directions and make sure you give your child the dosage appropriate for his age. Talk to your pediatrician about giving your child a daily multivitamin. A daily multivitamin will not harm your child, and can provide some peace of mind that your child is getting enough nutrients, even on days when he or she will eat nothing but bananas or peanut-butter-and-jelly sandwiches.

Food is strong medicine. Foods rich in certain vitamins or minerals and combined with nutrition supplements can be used to both prevent and treat a variety of common childhood illnesses and health problems. Though vitamins can be abused and overused to the point of causing adverse side effects, they can also be used safely and effectively.

How Much Is Too Much?

Though the body's demand for nutrients varies by age, sex, overall health, and activity level, the government has come up with general recommendations, known as the Recommended Dietary Allowances (RDAs), for the daily intake of key nutrients. These guidelines, developed by the Food and Nutrition Board of the National Research Council, list "adequate" levels of key nutrients. The RDAs are established with safety in mind: The amount is higher than the amount required for an average person to stay healthy, but lower than the amount that would cause the average person harm.

Despite these recommendations, a significant number of Americans—including those who are obese—fail to consume all the nutrients required for good health. That's not to say these people suffer from an obvious nutritional deficiency, but many do have a marginal deficiency that prevents them from functioning at an optimal level. In fact, government studies have shown that nearly half of all Americans have some kind of nutrient deficiency.

Faced with the possibility of nutritional shortfalls, some parents may be tempted to load up their children with vitamin and mineral supplements. But the "if some is good, more is better" approach does not apply to vitamins. Large doses of vitamins over long periods of time can trigger side effects, some of which can be serious.

Still, appropriate doses of vitamins *can* enhance your child's health. A study in the British medical journal *The Lancet* showed that regular use of a multiple vitamin-mineral supplement can increase the nonverbal intelligence of children. The study also discovered that a deficiency in any of the key essential nutrients can result in impaired brain and nervous system function.

Nutrition supplements can also help your child fight off illness: Vitamin C helps to prevent colds and reduce inflammation of the respiratory tract, beta-carotene helps heal mucous membranes and ward off infection, and vitamin E helps to heal the skin after sunburn, diaper rash, or other irritations.

A Primer on Key Nutrients

While there are more than forty vitamins and minerals known to be essential for human nutrition, we tend to focus on a handful of key nutrients. The table below summarizes the importance of these critical vitamins and minerals to your child's health.

Fat-Soluble Vitamins: These vitamins are stored in the body; mega-doses of these vitamins can build up in the body and cause dangerous side effects.

Vitamin A
What It Does: Promotes good night vision; aids in formation of teeth, bones, skin, hair, mucous membranes, and soft tissue; helps fight infection.
Warning Signs of Deficiency: Night blindness, slow or stunted growth in children, dry skin and eyes, increased susceptibility to infectious disease.
Signs of Overdose: Headaches, blurred vision, fatigue, diarrhea, joint pain, hair loss.
Good Food Sources: Carrots, sweet potatoes, kale, butternut squash, spinach, arugula, red bell peppers, dark green vegetables, liver, cheese.

Vitamin D
What It Does: Promotes the absorption of calcium, which is necessary for the development of bones and teeth; helps maintain proper blood levels of calcium and phosphorus.
Warning Signs of Deficiency: Soft bones, rickets.
Signs of Overdose: Calcium deposits in the heart, kidneys, and blood vessels; fragile bones; hypertension; high cholesterol; diarrhea.
Good Food Sources: Egg yolks, fish oil, fortified milk, butter, cheese, fortified cereals.

Vitamin E
What It Does: Helps in the formation of red blood cells, muscles, and other tissues; protects tissue against the damage of oxidation; assists in the utilization of vitamin K.

Warning Signs of Deficiency: Not known in humans.
Signs of Overdose: Headaches, excessive bleeding.
Good Food Sources: Poultry, seafood, seeds, nuts, wheat germ, eggs, vegetable oil, corn, olives, asparagus, green leafy vegetables.

Vitamin K

What It Does: Necessary for blood clotting and bone metabolism.
Warning Signs of Deficiency: Excessive bleeding, liver damage. (Deficiency is usually caused by an inability to absorb the vitamin, rather than an inadequate intake.)
Signs of Overdose: Jaundice in infants.
Good Food Sources: Spinach, leafy greens, oats, wheat bran, potatoes, cabbage, cauliflower, corn, soybeans.

Water-Soluble Vitamins: These vitamins are stored in smaller amounts in the body and therefore they should be consumed more often.

Vitamin B_1

What It Does: Helps cells convert carbohydrates into energy; essential for healthy brain and nerve cell function; promotes appetite.
Warning Signs of Deficiency: Fatigue, weakness, nerve damage, anxiety, hysteria, nausea, muscle cramps.
Signs of Overdose: Deficiency of other B vitamins; too much of one B vitamin may cause a deficiency of others.
Good Food Sources: Wheat germ, lean meats, fish, peas, dried beans, peanuts, fortified breads, pasta, cereals.

Vitamin B_6

What It Does: Helps maintain brain function; aids in the formation of red blood cells; essential to protein metabolism and absorption; helps with the synthesis of antibodies in the immune system.
Warning Signs of Deficiency: Depression, confusion, inflammation of mucous membranes of mouth, scaly skin, convulsions in infants.
Signs of Overdose: Numbness and neurological disorders.

Good Food Sources: Meats, fish, nuts, beans, bananas, eggs, whole grains, fortified cereals, spinach, potatoes, prunes.

Vitamin B_{12}

What It Does: Aids in the formation of red blood cells; helps maintain the central nervous system.

Warning Signs of Deficiency: Blood disorders and nerve damage.

Signs of Overdose: Rare; only in infants with genetic defect involving vitamin absorption.

Good Food Sources: Milk and milk products, eggs, meat, poultry, shellfish.

Folic Acid

What It Does: Necessary for formation of genetic material; helps produce red blood cells.

Warning Signs of Deficiency: Impaired cell division and abnormal red blood cells, anemia, diarrhea, bleeding gums, weight loss.

Signs of Overdose: Excess folic acid can interfere with zinc absorption, leading to slow wound healing and a weakened immune system.

Good Food Sources: Spinach, lentils, pinto beans, chickpeas, asparagus, beets, okra, broccoli, artichokes, citrus fruits, wheat bran. (Beginning in 1998, food manufacturers will add folic acid to enriched breads, flours, corn meals, pastas, rice, and other grain products.)

Vitamin C

What It Does: Helps promote healthy teeth and gums; aids in the absorption of iron; helps wounds heal; strengthens blood vessel walls.

Warning Signs of Deficiency: Bleeding gums, loose teeth, easy bruising, dry skin, loss of appetite.

Signs of Overdose: Kidney stones, urinary tract irritation, diarrhea.

Good Food Sources: Citrus fruits, red bell peppers, kale, kiwi fruit, broccoli, Brussels sprouts, cauliflower, strawberries, red cabbage, cantaloupe, potatoes.

Key Minerals Unlike vitamins, minerals are neither made nor broken down by the body. Many minerals are essential to body functions; however, they can cause adverse effects if you take too much of them.

Calcium
What It Does: Helps build and maintain strong bones and teeth; assists in the regulation of the heartbeat and other muscle contractions; necessary for blood clotting.
Warning Signs of Deficiency: Rickets, soft bones.
Signs of Overdose: Kidney stones and other calcium deposits in body tissues, mental confusion, lethargy.
Good Food Sources: Cheese, arugula, sardines and salmon (with bones), yogurt, kale, skim milk, dark green leafy vegetables.

Phosphorus
What It Does: Works with calcium to build and maintain bones and teeth; helps form cell membranes, DNA, and RNA.
Warning Signs of Deficiency: Weakness, bone pain.
Signs of Overdose: Low blood calcium levels, impaired use of iron and calcium.
Good Food Sources: Dairy products, egg yolks, meat, poultry, fish, legumes.

Magnesium
What It Does: Assists with metabolism and the formation of cells and genetic material; helps regulate normal heart rhythm.
Warning Signs of Deficiency: Cardiac arrhythmias; muscle weakness, twitching, cramps.
Signs of Overdose: Nervous system disorder, disruption in the calcium/magnesium balance.
Good Food Sources: Wheat bran, whole grains, dark green leafy vegetables, meat, milk, nuts, beans, bananas, apricots, beans, oysters, scallops.

Iron
What It Does: Helps in the formation of hemoglobin and myoglobin, both of which help carry oxygen through the blood.

Warning Signs of Deficiency: Weakness, fatigue, headache, shortness of breath, anemia.

Signs of Overdose: Diabetes, liver disease, cardiac arrhythmias. (WARNING: Iron poisoning is one of the most common causes of childhood poisoning deaths, primarily in young children who take their mothers' prenatal vitamins. As few as 6 high-potency iron tablets taken at one sitting can kill a 22-pound child.)

Good Food Sources: Clams, lentils, legumes, oats, oat bran, tofu, barley, beef, whole wheat bread, liver, fortified cereals.

Zinc

What It Does: Aids in wound healing; necessary for digestion, metabolism, and the functioning of the immune system.

Warning Signs of Deficiency: Slow wound healing, loss of appetite, slow or retarded growth.

Signs of Overdose: Nausea, vomiting, impaired immunity, high cholesterol, abdominal pain.

Good Food Sources: Oysters, pumpkin seeds, beef, pecans, cashews, lamb, almonds, turkey, sunflower seeds, wheat germ.

How Much Is Enough?

Therapeutic doses of vitamin and mineral supplements can be used for a limited time to give the body a boost in either preventing or managing an illness. To avoid overdose, give your child the age-appropriate dose for only the duration of the illness, or as long as recommended on the label. As the table on pages 14–15 shows, doses vary by age; after puberty, sex can affect dosage for certain nutrients.

	0 to 6 months	6 to 12 months	1–3 years	4–6 years	7–10 years	11–14 years male	11–14 years female	15–18 years male	15–18 years female
Vitamin A									
RDA[1]	1,000 IU[3]	2,000 IU	2,100 IU	2,000 IU	2,000 IU	2,500 IU	2,500 IU	5,000 IU	4,000 IU
Therapeutic Dose[2]	1,500 IU	2,500 IU	2,500 IU	2,500 IU	2,500 IU	3,000 IU	3,000 IU	3,000 IU	3,000 IU
Vitamin D									
RDA	200 IU	200 IU	400 IU	400 IU	400 IU	400 IU	400 IU	400 IU	400 IU
Therapeutic Dose	50 IU	50 IU	100 IU	100 IU	100 IU	100 IU	100 IU	100 IU	100 IU
Vitamin E									
RDA	3 mg	4 mg	6 mg	7 mg	7 mg	10 mg	8 mg	10 mg	8 mg
Therapeutic Dose	3 mg	5 mg	7 mg	8 mg	10 mg	15 mg	15 mg	20 mg	20 mg
Vitamin K									
RDA	5 mcg	10 mcg	15 mcg	20 mcg	30 mcg	45 mcg	45 mcg	65 mcg	55 mcg
Therapeutic Dose	3 mg	7 mg	10 mg	15 mg	20 mg	30 mg	30 mg	45 mg	45 mg
Vitamin C									
RDA	30 mg	35 mg	40 mg	45 mg	45 mg	50 mg	50 mg	60 mg	60 mg
Therapeutic Dose	40 mg	60 mg	100 mg	150 mg	200 mg	300 mg	300 mg	500 mg	500 mg
Vitamin B6									
RDA	0.3 mg	0.6 mg	1.0 mg	1.1 mg	1.4 mg	1.7 mg	1.4 mg	2.0 mg	1.5 mg
Therapeutic Dose	0.4 mg	0.6 mg	1.0 mg	1.0 mg	1.5 mg	2 mg	2 mg	2 mg	2 mg
Vitamin B12									
RDA	0.3 mg	0.5 mg	0.7 mg	1.0 mg	1.4 mg	2 mg	2 mg	2 mg	2 mg
Therapeutic Dose	1 mcg	2 mcg	2.5 mcg	3 mcg	4 mcg	5 mcg	5 mcg	5 mcg	5 mcg
Calcium									
RDA	400 mg	600 mg	800 mg	800 mg	800 mg	1,200 mg	1,200 mg	1,200 mg	1,200 mg
Therapeutic Dose	400 mg	500 mg	600 mg	700 mg	800 mg	1,000 mg	1,000 mg	1,200 mg	1,200 mg

	0 to 6 months	6 to 12 months	1–3 years	4–6 years	7–10 years	11–14 years male	11–14 years female	15–18 years male	15–18 years female
Magnesium									
RDA	40 mg	60 mg	80 mg	120 mg	170 mg	270 mg	280 mg	400 mg	300 mg
Therapeutic Dose	70 mg	90 mg	100 mg	200 mg	300 mg	400 mg	400 mg	400 mg	400 mg
Iron									
RDA	6 mg	10 mg	10 mg	10 mg	10 mg	12 mg	15 mg	12 mg	15 mg
Therapeutic Dose	10 mg	15 mg	15 mg	15 mg	12 mg	15 mg	18 mg	15 mg	18 mg
Zinc									
RDA	5 mg	5 mg	10 mg	10 mg	10 mg	15 mg	12 mg	15 mg	12 mg
Therapeutic Dose	4 mg	6 mg	10 mg	10 mg	10 mg	10 mg	10 mg	15 mg	15 mg

[1]RDA: Recommended Dietary Allowance
[2]Therapeutic Dose: Recommended dosage for nutrition supplements used for therapeutic reasons; higher doses should only be used for a limited time.
[3]IU: International Units

Treatment Tips

Whether you're giving a daily vitamin to maintain overall health, or using therapeutic doses to help manage a specific condition, keep these points in mind:

- Give your child vitamins and nutrition supplements with food, unless instructed otherwise on the product label.
- Store nutrition supplements away from heat and out of reach of your children. (Keep vitamins A and E in the refrigerator.)
- Throw away any vitamin or nutrition supplements that have passed their expiration date; these will not be as effective or potent as they should be.

··3··

Herbal Medicine:
Understanding Nature's
Medicines

Mother Nature is a pharmacist, and the leaves, bark, berries, flowers, seeds, and roots of plants are her drugs. Herbal medicines, or botanicals, can be used in the treatment of almost every childhood ailment, and they're often cheaper, safer, and more effective than synthetic drugs. Of course, herbal medicines cannot replace prescription and over-the-counter drugs, but they can complement conventional drug treatment in many cases.

Herbal medicines have a proven track record. Around the world, four out of five people use herbs as the basis of their medical care. European doctors often rely on herbal remedies, but herbs are not as widely used in the United States, in part because drug companies prefer to create synthetic medicines that can be patented and sold for a profit. The gifts of Mother Nature cannot be patented, so pharmaceutical companies prefer to produce and package synthetic drugs.

Despite the American preference for man-made medicines, about 25 percent of all prescription drugs in the U.S. contain active ingredients that come from plants. In a number of cases, drugs contain active ingredients that have been synthesized from chemicals similar to those that occur naturally in plants. For example, the herb ephedra contains ephedrine, a decongestant, and many allergy and cold-relief medications contain pseudoephedrine, a synthetic version of ephedrine.

Both pharmaceutical companies and modern herbalists owe a debt of gratitude to ancient herbalists who experimented with different plants and carefully monitored usage outcomes.

Based on experience, herbalists learned that some plants healed and others harmed. Today we understand the basics of biochemistry and why many herbal treatments work, but traditional herbal medicine is based on tens of thousands of years of trial and error. The tradition extends back before recorded history: A grave site of a Neanderthal man shows the use of yarrow, marsh mallow, and other healing herbs from 60,000 years ago.

Are Herbs Safe and Effective?

An alarming number of people hesitate before swallowing a couple of Tylenol but think nothing of taking a couple of capsules of an herbal remedy because they believe it is "natural" and therefore cannot harm them. While it's true that most herbs are safer than synthetic drugs and have fewer serious side effects, if used incorrectly, herbs can be as potent and as dangerous as prescription drugs. Some of the most toxic substances known come from plants. For example, the powerful rodent poison and central nervous system stimulant strychnine is derived from the plant *nux vomica*.

Unfortunately, herbal medicines can be misused easily. Unlike drugs, botanicals don't have to undergo rigorous testing or approval from the U.S. Food and Drug Administration before they wind up in health food stores. (The FDA classifies most herbal remedies as foods or food additives, rather than drugs.) That means it's up to the individual to know about the safety and efficacy of herbal treatments before using them or administering them to their children. It also means individuals should follow the package directions carefully when determining how much of an herbal treatment to take and whether it is safe for internal or external use. The absence of labeled warnings doesn't necessarily mean an herbal product is safe under all circumstances, so parents should proceed with caution.

Practicing Herbal Medicine

Herbal medicines come in a number of forms:

Tinctures are made by soaking an herb in a grain alcohol solution for a specified amount of time, usually several hours to several days, depending on the herb. The solution is then strained, yielding the tincture. (Tinctures also can be made using wine or apple cider vinegar instead of grain alcohol.)

Extracts are made by distilling off some of the alcohol, leaving behind a fluid with a higher concentration of the active ingredients. Most extracts are formed using vacuum distillation or filtration techniques, which do not require the use of high temperatures.

Capsules and tablets take the process one step further. They are solid extracts in which all the fluid is removed and the remaining concentrated solid is ground into granules or powders and shaped as capsules or tablets. If desired, the capsules can be opened and used to make infusions or compresses.

Teas are made by steeping or soaking herbs in boiling water for 5 minutes or so, then straining off the loose herbs. Teas should be made with 1 teaspoon of dried herb or 3 teaspoons of fresh herbs per cup of water.

Infusions are prepared like teas, but the herbs steep for 10–20 minutes, so the solution is darker, stronger, and usually more bitter.

Decoctions are basically infusions that are boiled instead of steeped; they are usually used for hard or woody herbs that include bark or roots.

Pellets are sugar-based granules that are usually taken sublingually.

Understanding Concentrations and Potency

The strength of potency of an herbal extract is expressed as a concentration in many cases. For example, an *extract* with a 4:1 concentration has one unit of extract derived from four units of herb. A *tincture* is usually a 1:10 concentration (10 units of tincture came from 1 unit of herbs). In general, a solid extract is at least four times as potent as an equal amount of fluid extract, and forty times as potent as a tincture, if they are produced from the same quality of herb.

Medicinal Herbs

Many herbs have healing properties that can be used to treat a variety of medical conditions. The table below lists the herbs used to treat the childhood illnesses described in this book, as well as their beneficial effects on the body and negative side effects. The table cannot identify every reported possible side effect of the herbs listed, but an effort has been made to highlight the most important. If you suspect that your child may be suffering from a side effect of an herb, contact a doctor as soon as possible. As noted in the table, some herbs can be taken internally, while others should be used externally (topically) to treat the conditions listed. Follow package instructions carefully.

Name	Used to treat	Beneficial effects	Possible side effects
Aloe vera (Use externally)	Athlete's foot Boils Burns Chicken pox Cuts, scrapes Frostnip Frostbite Marine stings Poison ivy Prickly heat	Promotes wound healing Kills bacteria	None known
Arnica (Use externally)	Muscle aches Sprains Sunburn	Kills bacteria Stimulates circulation	Skin rash
Basil (Use externally)	Acne	Kills bacteria on skin Stimulates immune system	None known

Name	Used to treat	Beneficial effects	Possible side effects
Black tea	Canker sores Cold sores Broken tooth Tooth decay	Eases breathing Prevents tooth decay Has astringent properties	Stomach upset
Calendula (Use externally)	Acne Burns Cradle cap Cuts, scrapes Dandruff Diaper rash Eczema Impetigo Prickly heat Spliers Tick bites	Kills germs Speeds tissue healing Reduces inflammation	None known
Cayenne pepper (Use externally)	Frostnip Frostbite	Stimulates circulation to skin's surface	Liver and kidney problems
Chamomile	Chicken pox Colds Colic Croup Headache Measles Mumps	Aids digestion Relieves anxiety Stimulates immune system	None known
Chickweed (Use externally)	Hives	Relieves skin irritation and inflammation	None known
Clove oil	Teething Toothache	Acts as an oral anesthetic Aids digestion Kills bacteria	Stomach upset
Coltsfoot	Cough	Soothes respiratory problems	Stomach upset

Name	Used to treat	Beneficial effects	Possible side effects
Comfrey (Use externally)	Insect bites Insect stings Sprains Sunburn	Promotes cell growth and wound healing Aids digestion	Liver damage
Dill	Gas	Relieves gas	Skin rash
Echinacea	Colds Earache Ear infection Flu Hoarseness Laryngitis Measles Roseola Sore throat Stuffy nose	Has antibiotic properties Stimulates immune system Promotes wound healing	Tingling on tongue
Ephedra	Allergies	Clears congestion	Increases blood pressure Insomnia Dry mouth
Eucalyptus (Use externally)	Fever Heatstroke	Has expectorant properties Kills bacteria	Deadly if used internally
Evening primrose oil (Use externally or internally)	Eczema	Soothes the skin	Headache Skin rash Nausea
Eyebright (Use externally)	Pinkeye	Soothes sore, itching eye Controls fever	None known
Fennel	Colic Gas	Soothes stomach and digestive problems	Skin irritation Nausea Vomiting
Fenugreek (Use externally)	Splinters	Draws foreign objects to skin's surface	None known

Name	Used to treat	Beneficial effects	Possible side effects

Garlic	Allergies
	Animal bites
	Athlete's foot
	Colds
	Cold sores
	Earache
	Ear infection
	Fever
	Flu
	Food poisoning
	Gas
	Lice
	Pinworms
	Runny nose
	Sore throat
	Stuffy nose
	Urinary tract
	  infection
		Has antibiotic
		  and antiseptic
		  properties
		Expels worms
		Lowers blood
		  pressure
		Decreases
		  cholesterol
			Nausea
			Gas

Ginger	Boils
	Dizziness
	Fever
	Flu
	Food poisoning
	Gas
	Headache
	Stomachache
	Vomiting
		Aids digestion
		Promotes
		  perspiration
		Relieves fever
		Eases motion
		  sickness
			Diarrhea
			Heartburn

Goldenseal
  (Use externally
  or internally)
	Animal bites
	Boils
	Canker sores
	Diarrhea
	Flu
	Impetigo
	Lice
	Measles
	Roseola
	Sore throat
	Stuffy nose
		Has antibiotic
		  properties
		Fights infection
		Stimulates
		  immune
		  system
		Aids digestion
			Vomiting
			Diarrhea

Jewelweed
  (Use externally)
	Poison ivy	Soothes
		  dermatitis
			None known

Name	Used to treat	Beneficial effects	Possible side effects
Lavender (Use externally)	Burns Heatstroke	Soothes burns and stings Kills bacteria Promotes healing	None known
Licorice	Canker sores Colds Constipation Cough Stomachache Vomiting	Soothes respiratory tract Kills bacteria	High blood pressure
Lungwort	Cough	Has expectorant properties	None known
Marjoram	Cold sores	Aids digestion Inhibits growth of Herpes simplex	None known
Mullein	Cough	Has expectorant properties Acts as a sedative	None known
Myrrh	Boils	Has astringent properties Kills bacteria	Diarrhea
Oatmeal (Use externally)	Chicken pox Eczema Measles Roseola	Eases itching	None known
Parsley	Bad breath	Has diuretic properties Reduces fever Freshens breath	Skin rash Headache

Name	Used to treat	Beneficial effects	Possible side effects
Peppermint	Colic Diarrhea Gas Heatstroke Mumps Muscle aches Vomiting	Aids digestion Reduces fever Relieves gas and diarrhea	Stomach irritation
Psyllium	Constipation	Absorbs fluid in the intestines	Stomach upset

Rosemary	Dandruff
	Diarrhea
		Reduces muscle
		  spasms
		Increases
		  circulation
			Nausea
			Diarrhea

Skullcap	Headache	Acts as a sedative	Irregular heartbeat

Slippery elm
(Not for internal use)
	Hoarseness
	Laryngitis
	Splinters
		Soothes throat
		  when used as
		  a gargle
			None known

Tea tree oil (Use externally)	Acne Animal bites Athlete's foot Boils Burns Impetigo Insect bites Insect stings Lice Marine stings Ringworm Teething Tick bites	Kills germs	None known

Thyme	Allergies
	Bronchitis
	Dandruff
		Has antiseptic
		  properties
		Clears
		  congestion
		Aids digestion
			Diarrhea
			Skin rash

Uva ursi	Urinary tract infection	Has astringent
		  properties
		Decongestant
		Aids digestion
			Urine dark
			  green
			Vomiting

Name	Used to treat	Beneficial effects	Possible side effects
Witch hazel	Prickly heat	Has astringent properties	None known
Wormwood*	Pinworms	Stimulates appetite Expels worms Reduces fever	Uterine contractions Birth defects

*Use only under a doctor's supervision

How Much Is Enough?

The appropriate dose of herbal remedies taken internally varies by age. Herbs used in external treatments do not vary by age.

Birth to 2 years*	2 years to 6 years	6 years to 12 years	12 years to Adult
3 drops of tincture diluted in ¼ cup of water	10 drops of tincture diluted in ¼ cup of water	15 drops of tincture	25 drops of tincture
3 teaspoons of tea	¼ cup of tea	½ cup of tea	1 cup of tea
Do not use capsules or tablets	Do not use capsules or tablets	1 capsule or tablet	2 capsules or tablets

*An infant can also receive herbal treatment through breast milk: If a breast-feeding mother takes the adult dose of an herbal remedy, the appropriate dose of herbs will be passed on to the baby.

Treatment Tips

- If the herb has a strong and unpleasant taste, dilute it in water or apple juice.
- Always start with the lowest possible dose or frequency and give more of a drug if necessary.
- Look for side effects: Keep an eye out for nausea, diarrhea, or headache within an hour or two of giving your child any

herb. If your child experiences a severe reaction, call the doctor immediately.

- Don't use herbal ointments or topical treatments on broken skin, unless directed.

··4··

Homeopathy:
Using Natural
Solutions

In the past few years, a growing number of Americans have
been reconsidering the traditional high-tech approach to healing and turning to low-tech, natural treatments for a number
of common ailments. One increasingly popular option: homeopathy.

The practice of homeopathy was developed in the early
nineteenth century by Dr. Samuel Hahnemann (1755–1843), a
German physician who had been trained in conventional medicine. During his career, Dr. Hahnemann became disillusioned
with the crude and sometimes harmful medical practices of the
day, which included bloodletting, induced vomiting, and the
use of massive doses of (poorly understood) drugs. Hahnemann developed homeopathy in response to these harsh ex-
cesses of orthodox medicine.

Hahnemann believed in the healing powers of nutrition and
exercise—radical ideas at the time—and he experimented with
other methods of treatment, usually testing potential remedies
on himself. In one experiment, Hahnemann tested cinchona
(also known as Peruvian bark), which is the natural source of
quinine. When he took small doses of cinchona, Hahnemann
developed the symptoms of malaria: fever, chills, thirst, and a
pounding headache. He believed that cinchona would be effective in treating malaria because of its ability to produce
similar symptoms to those of the disease.

The results of this experiment led to Hahnemann's first theory, the Law of Similars, or "like cures like." According

to the theory, certain illnesses can be cured by giving the sick person minuscule doses of natural substances—plants, minerals, chemicals, and animal substances—that would produce the symptoms of the disease in a healthy person.

In further experiments, Hahnemann learned that higher concentrations of substances caused more side effects, but he could dilute a medication and still preserve its healing powers through a pharmacological process he called "potentization." Hahnemann found that by repeatedly diluting a substance with distilled water or alcohol and shaking it vigorously between each dilution, he could increase the potency of the medicine. These findings resulted in Hahnemann's theory, the Law of Infinitesimals, which states that the smaller the dose of active ingredient, the more potent the cure.

Homeopathy was put to the test in dealing with epidemic diseases, such as cholera, typhoid, yellow fever, and scarlet fever. The success of the treatment led to widespread interest in its practice. The first homeopathy college opened in Philadelphia in 1836, and eight years later a group of homeopaths formed the American Institute of Homeopathy, the first national medical organization in the country. By the end of the nineteenth century, there were fifteen thousand homeopaths and twenty-two schools of homeopathy nationwide. Homeopathy also flourished and continues to thrive in Europe, particularly in Great Britain, where the Queen of England has her own homeopathic physician and the British National Health Service covers homeopathic procedures.

In the United States, however, homeopathy rapidly fell out of favor. At the end of the nineteenth century, one out of every five American doctors practiced homeopathy, but by the middle of the twentieth century the American practice of homeopathy had all but disappeared. The discovery of antibiotics and other advances in modern medicine lured people to support a more "scientific" approach to healing. Professional medical groups, influenced by these developments, began to expel physicians who practiced homeopathy or consulted with homeopaths.

Only recently has the homeopathic revival begun in the United States, in part because skeptics have been quieted by a number of studies showing that homeopathic remedies do help in the healing process. In 1991, the *British Medical Journal* tried to put the question to rest by publishing an analysis of 107 clinical studies involving the efficacy of homeopathy. Out of the total, 81 of the studies showed that the homeopathic treatment was more effective than a placebo.

No one knows exactly why homeopathy works, but some experts theorize that the repeated dilution and shaking establishes a certain electrochemical pattern in the water. Then, when someone takes a homeopathic remedy, the electrochemical pattern in the remedy affects the electrochemical pattern of the water in the human body. Other experts suggest that the potentization changes the electromagnetic fields in the body in some subtle way. Both of these theories involve energy changes at a subatomic level, a level that we can never see and few of us will ever understand.

Additional research will undoubtedly be conducted to prove or disprove various theories about homeopathy. In the meantime, homeopaths and open-minded parents will continue to use the treatments, not because they understand how they work but because they know that they do.

Treat the Person, Not the Disease

Homeopaths and traditional doctors approach healing from different points of view. Homeopaths believe illness is not localized in one organ or manifested in one symptom, so when prescribing treatment they consider the entire person, both mind and body. Practitioners of conventional medicine, on the other hand, tend to focus on suppressing symptoms, taking little or no account of the person's emotional or overall physical condition. Homeopaths consider physical symptoms as positive signs that the body is hard at work defending and healing itself. Rather than trying to eliminate symptoms, homeopathic remedies sometimes even aggravate symptoms for a time as they stimulate the body's self-healing mechanism.

Because homeopaths prescribe treatments based on a variety of very specific symptoms reported by the patient, the home use of homeopathic remedies should be limited to treatment of relatively minor ailments, such as colds, runny noses, and other nonlife-threatening conditions. If your child experiences recurrent or potentially dangerous symptoms, consider consulting with a trained homeopath.

A visit to a homeopath usually starts out with a long interview, including detailed questions about your child's medical history, as well as information on your child's overall energy, sensitivity to temperature and water, sleep habits, food preferences, and emotional state. All of these factors must be taken into account by a homeopath when deciding which of more than two thousand remedies to prescribe.

Practicing Homeopathy

Unlike other medical practices, the selection of the appropriate homeopathic remedy varies from patient to patient, depending on the patient profile and the specific symptoms that are present. For example, two children might pass a cold virus from one to the other, but the children would receive different treatments, based on their individual symptoms.

Homeopathic remedies are prepared according to standards of the United States Homeopathy Pharmacopoeia and come in a variety of potencies, based on the strength of dilution. The three most common forms of remedies are the mother tincture, x potencies, and c potencies:

The mother tincture. The mother tincture is an alcohol-based extract of a specific substance, such as the plant Yellow Jasmine or the mineral potassium carbonate. They are usually used topically.

X potencies. The x represents the Roman numeral 10. In homeopathic remedies with x potencies the mother tincture has been diluted to 1 part in 10 (1 drop of tincture to every 9 drops of alcohol). The number before the x tells how many times the mother tincture has been diluted. For example, a 12x potency represents 12 dilutions of 1 in 10. The more the substance is diluted, the more potent it becomes, so a remedy with a 30x potency is considered stronger or more potent than one with a 12x potency.

C potencies. The c represents the Roman number 100, so homeopathy remedies with a c potency have been diluted to

1 part in 100 (1 drop of tincture to every 99 drops of alcohol), making them much stronger than x potencies. Again, the number before the c represents the number of dilutions. A 3c potency represents a substances that has been diluted to one part in 100 three times; by the time 3c is reached, the dilution is 1 part per million. In general, 6c is the potency recommended for most acute or self-limiting ailments, and 30c for chronic conditions or emergencies.

When you use the right remedy, it will work quickly and you can discontinue treatment. The wrong remedy will cause no harm, but your child's condition will not improve. Because the amount of active ingredient is so small, side effects from homeopathic remedies are virtually nonexistent, even among infants.

Common Homeopathic Remedies

Homeopathic remedies come in pellet, tablet, and liquid form. Pellets and tablets are the best forms to administer to children—and most kids love them because they consist primarily of sugar. Avoid touching them, though. Instead, shake the pellets into a measuring spoon and place them under your child's tongue and allow them to dissolve. Homeopathic tinctures (liquid remedies) aren't recommended for children because of their high alcohol content. Homeopathic creams, ointments, and salves can be made by mixing diluted remedies with cream or gel base for topical use.

Common Name	Latin Name	Made From	Used For
Aconite	*Aconitum napellus*	Wolfsbane, blue aconite	Asthma Colds Concussion Croup Fever Mumps Pinkeye Stomachache Teething
Actaea	*Actaea spicata*	baneberry, herb Christopher	Teething

Common Name	Latin Name	Made From	Used For
Aethusa	*Aethusa cynapium*	Fool's parsley	Hiccups
Allium	*Allium cepa*	Red onion	Colds
Alumina	*Alumina*	Aluminum oxide	Constipation
Antimonium	*Antimonium crudum*	Black sulfide of antimony	Impetigo
Antimonium tart.	*Antimonium tartaricum*	Potassium antimony tartrate	Cough
Apis	*Apis mellifica*	Honey bees	Frostbite Hives Prickly heat
Argentum nit.	*Argentum nitricum*	Silver nitrate	Pinkeye
Arnica	*Arnica montana*	Leopard's band, Fallkraut	Black eye Bruises Burns Concussion Cuts Hoarseness Insect bites Nosebleeds Sprains Tooth broken
Arsenicum	*Arsenicum album*	Arsenic trioxide	Asthma Dandruff Diarrhea Flu Impetigo Vomiting
Aurum	*Aurum metallicum*	Gold	Bad breath
Baptisia	*Baptisia tinctoria*	Wild indigo	Food poisoning

Common Name	Latin Name	Made From	Used For
Belladonna	*Atropa belladonna*	Deadly nightshade	Boils Chicken pox Cough Earache Fever Heatstroke Measles Mumps Roseola Sore throat Stuffy nose
Bryonia	*Bryonia alba*	White bryony	Bronchitis Sprains
Calcarea	*Calcarea carbonica*	Calcium carbonate from oyster shells	Diarrhea Dizziness Tooth decay
Calcarea phos.	*Calcarea phosphorica*	Calcium phosphate	Anemia Bed-wetting
Calcarea sulph.	*Calcarea sulphurica*	Gypsum, calcium sulfate	Acne
Cantharis	*Cantharis lytta vesicatoria*	Spanish fly	Insect bites Urinary tract infection
Capsicum	*Capsicum annuum*	Cayenne pepper	Cold sores
Carbo veg.	*Carbo vegetabilis*	Vegetable charcoal made from beech, birch, or poplar wood	Asthma Colic
Carbolic ac.	*Carbolicum acidum*	Carbolic acid, phenol	Insect bites
Causticum	*Causticum hahnemanni*	Potassium hydrate	Bed-wetting
Chamomilla	*Chamomilla vulgaris*	German chamomile	Colic Teething
Cina	*Cina artemisia maritima*	Sea southernwood, wormseed	Pinworms

Common Name	Latin Name	Made From	Used For
Coffea	*Coffea cruda*	Unroasted coffee	Toothache
Colocynth	*Citrullus colocynthis*	Bitter apple	Colic Food poisoning
Conium	*Conium maculatum*	Hemlock	Dizziness
Crotalus	*Crotalus horridus*	Rattlesnake venom	Insect bites
Cuprum	*Cuprum metallicum*	Copper	Heatstroke
Equisetum	*Equisetum byemale*	Scouring rush, horsetail	Bed-wetting
Euphatorium	*Eupatorium perfoliatum*	Boneset, thoroughwort	Flu
Euphrasia	*Euphrasia officinalis*	Eyebright	Colds Measles
Ferrum phos.	*Ferrum phosphoricum*	Iron phosphate	Croup Sore throat Sunburn
Gelsemium	*Gelsemium sempervirens*	Yellow jasmine	Colds Dizziness Fever Headache Measles
Graphites	*Graphites*	Black lead from pencils	Cradle cap Eczema
Hepar sulph.	*Hepar sulphuris calcareum*	Calcium sulfide	Acne Boils Burns Earache
Hydrastis	*Hydrastis canadensis*	Goldenseal	Runny nose
Ignatia	*Ignatia amara*	St. Ignatius' bean	Stomachache
Ipecac	*Cephaelis ipecacuanha*	Ipecacuanha	Bronchitis Nosebleeds Vomiting
Iris	*Iris versicolor*	Blue flag	Headache

Common Name	Latin Name	Made From	Used For
Kali bichrom.	*Kali bichromicum*	Potassium bichromate	Bronchitis Burns Stuffy nose
Kali carb.	*Kali carbonicum*	Potassium carbonate	Asthma
Kali mur.	*Kali muriaticum*	Potassium chloride	Croup Warts
Lachesis	*Trigonocepha-lus lachesis*	Bushmaster snake venom	Frostbite
Ledum	*Ledum palustre*	Wild rosemary	Black eye Bruises
Lycopdium	*Lycopodium clavatum*	Wolfsclaw club moss	Constipation
Magnesia phos.	*Magnesia phosphorica*	Magnesium phosphate	Diarrhea
Mercurius	*Mercurius solubilis hahnemanni*	Mercury	Chicken pox Flu
Mezereum	*Daphne mezereum*	Spurge olive, mezereon	Eczema Impetigo
Myristica	*Myristica sebifera*	Ucuuba tree	Boils
Natrum carb.	*Natrum carbonicum*	Sodium carbonate	Warts
Natrum mur.	*Natrum muriaticum*	Salt, sodium chloride	Headache Runny nose
Nux	*Strychnos nux vomica*	Poison nut tree	Bad breath Constipation Dizziness Hiccups Stomachache
Phosphoric ac.	*Phosphoricum acidum*	Phosphoric acid	Food poisoning
Phosphorus	*Phosphorus*	Phosphous	Fever Hoarseness Nosebleeds Sore throat
Phytolacca	*Phytolacca decandra*	Poke root	Mumps Roseola Sore throat

Common Name	Latin Name	Made From	Used For
Pilocarpin mur.	*Pilocarpin muriaticum*	Hydrochlorate or pilocarpine	Mumps
Plantago	*Plantago major*	Ribwort, great plantain	Toothache
Pulsatilla	*Pulsatilla nigricans*	Wind flower	Bad breath Bronchitis Chicken pox Cough Diarrhea Earache Measles Mumps Pinkeye Runny nose Vomiting
Rhus tox.	*Rhus toxicodendron*	Poison ivy	Chicken pox Cold sores Diaper rash Eczema Hives Poison ivy Sprains
Ruta	*Ruta graveolens*	Rue	Bruises
Sanguinaria	*Sanguinaria canadensis*	Bloodroot	Runny nose
Sepia	*Sepia officialis*	Cuttlefish ink	Dandruff
Silicea	*Silicea terra*	Flint	Acne Boils Splinters Stuffy nose Tooth decay
Sol	*Sol*	Sugar water exposed to sunlight	Sunburn
Spongia	*Spongia tosta*	Roasted common sponge	Cough Hoarseness
Staphisagria	*Delphinium staphisagria*	Stavesacre	Cuts

Common Name	Latin Name	Made From	Used For
Sulphur	*Sulphur*	Sublimated sulphur	Acne Chicken pox Dandruff Diaper rash Eczema Measles Ringworm Warts
Tellurium	*Tellurium*	Tellurium	Ringworm
Thuja	*Thuja occidentalis*	White cedar	Athlete's foot
Urtica	*Urtica wrens*	Small nettle	Burns Hives
Viola	*Viola tricolor*	Pansy	Cradle cap

Treatment Tips

- Give your child a homeopathic remedy at least a half hour before or after eating. Strong flavors can decrease the effectiveness of the remedies since the impact of the homeopathic remedy is very subtle. Odors can also affect efficacy; if possible, avoid strong smells, such as perfumes, chemical odors, and other scents, for a half hour before or after taking a homeopathic remedy.
- Know when to quit. If you give a treatment for a condition that clears up in 15 minutes, you don't need to give another dose. If the symptom later returns, you can administer a second dose. Should the second attempt also fail, contact a homeopath or your pediatrician.

··5··

Acupressure: The Healing Touch

Acupressure is an ancient Chinese healing art that uses touch to stimulate the body's natural healing in the same way that acupuncture uses fine needles to activate the same points. Acupressure involves using the fingers to apply pressure to key "points," which in turn eases muscular tension and increases blood circulation to the pressured spots. This combination of deep relaxation and improved circulation promotes healing and helps ease secondary symptoms, such as back pain or difficulty breathing caused by tension. The techniques are safe and effective (as long as you follow certain basic rules), and they can be done by almost anyone, anytime, anywhere.

Most people use some acupressure without realizing it: Do you massage your temples when you have a headache? And do you instinctively rub an injury, such as a bruised shin when you knock it on the coffee table? These reflexive responses can be thought of as simple acupressure techniques. In fact, the art of acupressure evolved from these basic touching instincts.

At least 5,000 years ago, the Chinese observed that pressing certain points on the body helped to relieve pain in other parts of the body. Over the centuries, these healers used trial and error to establish and refine an intricate network of pressure points that is the foundation for the practice of acupressure today.

This time-honored technique has been used with success in Asian cultures for thousands of years. Acupressure works on both children and adults and can help relieve a number of common childhood ailments, such as constipation, bedwetting, nausea, and gas. Of course, acupressure cannot replace traditional medical care, but it can add an important new dimension to it. Besides, even if your child's condition does not improve following the treatment, a gentle massage by a loving parent surely won't hurt.

How It Works

Acupressure points are spots on the body that are particularly sensitive to the bioelectrical impulses associated with touch. These points lie along pathways through the body that carry "life energy" (this energy is called *Qi* or *Chi* in China, *Ki* in Japan, and *Prana* in India). The energy flows smoothly in active and healthy children, but it is blocked or deficient in a child who is sick or injured. Stimulating these points—either with finger pressure (acupressure) or needles (acupuncture)—unlocks the flow of energy and releases the body's natural pain-relieving chemicals, endorphins, into the bloodstream. In addition to easing pain, the stimulation increases blood flow to the area, causing the surrounding muscles to relax and promoting healing.

Pressure points work in several ways. When you press a point where the pain or disorder occurs, you are stimulating a *local point*. When applying pressure to a point that affects a distant part of the body, you are activating a *trigger point*. Trigger points work through a network of electrical channels called *meridians* that run along each side of the body; there are twelve major meridians, each named after or corresponding to a different organ. The meridians connect the acupressure points throughout the body, a sort of electrical wiring system that carries the life energy responsible for physical, emotional, and spiritual health. Because acupressure points are connected through this network, stimulating one point can carry messages to other parts of the body.

The acupressure points referred to in this book include both local points and trigger points, depending on the condition being treated. While you may find it more intuitively appro-

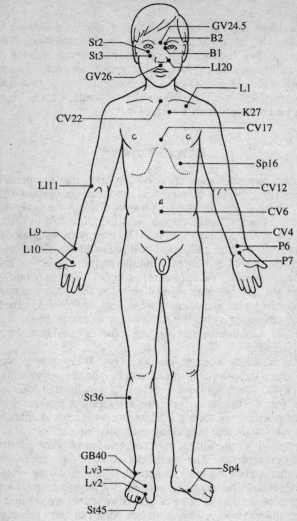

KEY:
B   Bladder   GV   Governing Vessel
CV   Conception Vessel   L   Lung
GB   Gall Bladder   LI   Large Intestine

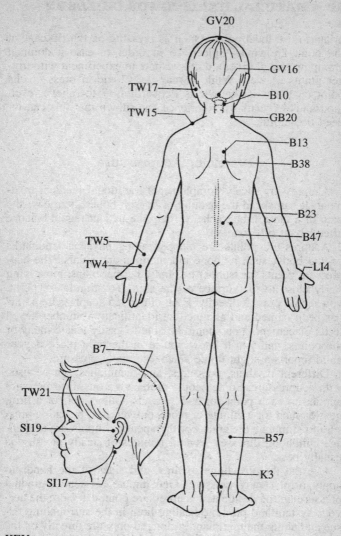

KEY:

LV	Liver	Sp	Spleen
P	Pericardium	St	Stomach
SI	Small Intestine	TW	Triple Warmer

priate to use local points (such as pressing on the rib cage at the point known as Spleen 16 in order to ease abdominal cramping and diarrhea), don't hesitate to experiment with trigger points as well. While it may defy logic to press on the point on the wrist known as Pericardium 7 to relieve fever, thousands of years of experience has shown that this can indeed be helpful.

Practicing Acupressure

Acupressure nicely complements traditional medical treatment. It can speed the healing of broken bones, help ease the pain of a tension headache, or help the patient regain balance after a bout of dizziness.

Acupressure points are mapped along physical landmarks on the body, such as bone indentations and joints. The acupressure points (or tsubos) lie along the meridians, most lying fairly close to the surface of the skin. To stimulate a point, you should press it directly. Each of the 365 acupressure points has been named and assigned an identification number keyed to its placement. You should be able to easily locate many of the points, and you'll know you're in the right place if your child reports a slight tingle when you apply pressure.

Different rhythms, pressures, and techniques can be used with acupressure. Some people prefer vigorous, firm pressure applied to each point for 3–5 seconds. Others opt for a firm, gentle touch for a minute or more, or even fast, pulsating pressure to stimulate the area. For therapeutic acupressure to manage childhood illnesses, several minutes of steady pressure is usually best.

Use the thumbs, finger, palms, and sides of the hands to apply firm, steady pressure. One minute of steady, gradual pressure on the designated acupressure point can calm the nervous system and promote healing both in the surrounding tissue and along the meridian. Prolonged pressure directly on the point for approximately 3 minutes is ideal. Each point will feel different when pressed; some will feel tense, others sore and achy. Don't press so hard that your child complains, but apply enough force to stimulate the point.

Whenever possible, apply pressure with the middle finger. You may want to massage or rub the area, but it's best to hold the point steady with a slow, firm pressure, while holding the finger at a right angle to the body. Begin by stimulating the point with a light touch, then gradually increase the force until a deep, constant pressure is achieved. Don't jab the skin; apply and release the pressure gradually and steadily. If possible, work the left and right sides of the body at the same time. If your hand gets tired, ease up on the point, shake out your hand and try again. Hold for a few minutes until you feel a regular pulse or until any soreness disappears, then gradually release the pressure.

When starting out, you may only be able to practice acupressure for several minutes at a time. Even after you have built up your "finger" strength, you should never hold a single pressure point for longer than 5 or 10 minutes. Do not work any area of the body, such as the face or back, for longer than 15 minutes.

While practicing acupressure, have your child perform deep breathing to keep her body fully oxygenated, and to help the acupressure in releasing the pain and tension. Breathe slowly and deeply along with your child; it will help you and your child to focus and concentrate on the healing process.

Name of Point	Location of Point	Pressure Point Used to Treat These Conditions
Abdominal Sorrow	Spleen 16	Abdominal cramping Colic Diarrhea Hiccups Nausea
Active Pond	Triple Warmer 4	Fever Wrist pain
Big Mound	Pericardium 7	Fever Wrist pain

Name of Point	Location of Point	Pressure Point Used to Treat These Conditions
Bigger Rushing	Liver 3	Allergies Canker sores Congestion Diaper rash Headache Pinkeye
Bigger Stream	Kidney 3	Bed-wetting Earache Incontinence Urinary tract infection
Center of Power	Conception Vessel 12	Hiccups
Crooked Pond	Large Intestine 11	Allergies Constipation Fever Hoarseness Insect bites Itching
Drilling Bamboo	Bladder 2	Headaches Sinus pain Stuffy nose
Ear Gate	Triple Warmer 21	Earache
Elegant Mansion	Kidney 27	Coughing Hiccups Hoarseness Sore throat
Eyes Bright	Bladder 1	Nosebleed Pinkeye
Facial Beauty	Stomach 3	Acne Nosebleed Stuffy nose Teething pain

Name of Point	Location of Point	Pressure Point Used to Treat These Conditions
Fish Border	Lung 10	Asthma Breathing problems Coughing
Four Whites	Stomach 2	Acne
Gate Origin	Conception Vessel	Incontinence
Gates of Consciousness	Gallbladder 20	Dizziness Headache Runny nose Stuffy nose
Grandfather Grandson	Spleen 4	Diarrhea Gas Indigestion Stomachache Vomiting
Great Abyss	Lung 9	Asthma Coughing Itching
Heaven Rushing Out	Conception Vessel 22	Bronchitis Coughing Sore throat
Heavenly Appearance	Small Intestine 17	Bruises Hives
Heavenly Pillar	Bladder 10	Acne Anxiety Eczema Sore throat
Heavenly Rejuvenation	Triple Warmer 15	Anxiety Cold symptoms Flu symptoms
Inner Gate	Pericardium 6	Croup Nausea Vomiting

Name of Point	Location of Point	Pressure Point Used to Treat These Conditions
Joining the Valley	Large Intestine 4	Allergies Black eye pain Constipation Flu symptoms Headache Itching Nosebleed Sore throat Stuffy nose Teething pain
Letting Go	Lung 1	Asthma Breathing problems Bronchitis Coughing Hiccups
Listening Place	Small Intestine 19	Earache Teething pain
Lung Associated	Bladder 13	Asthma Breathing problems Coughing
Middle of a Person	Governing Vessel 26	Dizziness Hay fever Muscle cramps Nosebleed
One Hundred Meeting Point	Governing Vessel 20	Headache caused by heatstroke
Outer Gate	Triple Warmer 5	Anxiety
Penetrate Heaven	Bladder 7	Congestion Headache
Sea of Energy	Conception Vessel 6	Allergies Colic Constipation Diarrhea Dizziness Gas

Name of Point	Location of Point	Pressure Point Used to Treat These Conditions
Sea of Tranquility	Conception Vessel 17	Chest tension Croup
Sea of Vitality	Bladder 23, Bladder 47	Acne Black eye Bruises Dizziness Eczema
Severe Mouth	Stomach 45	Food poisoning Nausea Stomachache
Supporting Mountain	Bladder 57	Muscles aches Stomachache
Third Eye Point	Governing Vessel 24.5	Cold symptoms Dizziness Headache
Three Mile Point	Stomach 36	Acne Bruises Colic Constipation Eczema Gas Hives Nausea Stomachache Vomiting
Travel Between	Liver 2	Diarrhea Nausea Stomachache Vomiting
Vital Diaphragm	Bladder 38	Breathing problems Bronchitis Coughing
Welcoming Perfume	Large Intestine 20	Congestion Runny nose Sinus pain

Name of Point	Location of Point	Pressure Point Used to Treat These Conditions
Wilderness Mound	Gallbladder 40	Ankle sprains
Wind Mansion	Governing Vessel 16	Flu symptoms Headache Nosebleed Sore throat
Wind Screen	Triple Warmer 17	Acne Earache Hiccups Hives Sore throat Teething pain

Treatment Tips

- Make sure your hands are clean and warm before touching your child.
- Keep your fingernails short to avoid scratching or poking your child.
- Before you begin, ask your child to relax and take a few deep breaths. This moment of relaxation will help your child focus on her body and the healing process.
- Never jab or poke a pressure point. Apply steady pressure with gradually increasing force for the first 30 seconds or so, hold steady for 1–3 minutes, then gradually ease up on the pressure during the final 30 seconds or so. Avoid any abrupt motions.
- Stop pressing any time your child complains that the touch is painful. Acupressure should not hurt.
- Press gently on the lymph areas, including the groin, throat, and armpits.
- Never press an area that has been burned, bruised, cut, sprained, or infected. However, you can press points near

the injured area to increase blood circulation and release muscular tension.

- Don't work on a freshly scarred area. Again, you can apply pressure several inches away from the injury to help heal the area, but not directly on the injury.

· PART 2 ·

Natural Healing from A to Z

Acne

The teenage years can be tough on both you and your child. You have to put up with your child's emotional roller-coaster rides and attitude problems, but your child must endure the worst curse of all: Acne.

Acne starts deep in the pores of the skin, where the sebaceous glands produce sebum, a concoction of oils and waxes designed to keep the skin moist and lubricated. As any acne-prone adolescent can tell you, the sebaceous glands are concentrated in the face, back, chest, and shoulders—the same areas that tend to break out most often.

During puberty, the body produces testosterone and other hormones that increase the production of sebum. (Both males and females produce testosterone, though males usually have more of it.) The excess sebum blocks the pores, causing blackheads. When bacteria grow beneath the skin and release enzymes that break down the sebum, the result is whiteheads or pimples.

Kids with problem acne tend to have higher levels of 5-alpha-reductase, an enzyme that converts testosterone to dihydrotestosterone (or DHT), which seems to stimulate acne. Because of these hormonal links, acne usually shows up around age 14 for girls and 16 for boys, and starts to fade by the early 20s.

But acne isn't restricted to adolescence; it can last well into adulthood. Even babies can experience "infantile" acne, breakouts caused by hormonal fluctuations taking place as the newborn adjusts to life outside of mommy's womb. (These breakouts usually last only a week or so, and they don't require treatment.)

Unfortunately, there isn't much you can do to prevent acne, though you can try to reassure your child that the condition isn't his fault. Acne isn't caused by dirt or poor hygiene; the pimples form beneath the surface of the skin, so no amount of scrubbing can prevent them entirely. Most likely your child is going to have to learn to live with acne (at least for a few years), but there are ways of making that time easier for him—and you.

Traditional Treatments

You are what you eat. Some foods trigger acne, but there is confusion over exactly which foods to blame. There was a time when fatty foods were considered the culprits, but the latest thinking is that iodine, which is added to salt, is the true troublemaker. With this in mind, you should encourage your child to avoid salty foods such as chips, burgers, and highly processed foods. Also, remind your child to eat plenty of foods that fortify the skin, such as those rich in beta-carotene (sweet potatoes, dark green leafy vegetables, and apricots), zinc (oysters, wheat germ, beans), and acidophilus (yogurt).

Forget the chocolate myth. Many adolescents, and some of their doctors, believe that chocolate exacerbates breakouts. Fortunately for die-hard chocoholics, this simply isn't true. Dermatologists conducted a study on 65 adolescents willing to eat the equivalent of one pound of chocolate a day for a month. The findings: Chocolate had no bearing on the complexion.

Zap those zits. Over-the-counter acne lotions and gels containing benzoyl peroxide help dry out pimples and avoid new breakouts when used following package directions. Be patient; it usually takes at least 6–8 weeks to see noticeable results. WARNING: Some people are allergic to benzoyl peroxide, so before having your child slather it all over his face, encourage him to test a dab on the inside of his forearm. If the area does not shows signs of irritation within 24 hours after administering, it should be safe to use. If the area looks red or burned, ask a dermatologist to recommend another product.

Start out small. Different acne products contain different concentrations of active ingredients. Have your child start out with a product containing only 2.5 percent benzoyl peroxide, then turn to the more potent 5 and 10 percent solutions if the lower dosage doesn't clear the acne within a month or so. Keep in mind, though, the higher the concentration, the more likely the lotion will irritate the skin, causing redness and dry patches.

Watch where you're putting that. Benzoyl peroxide not only clears acne, it also bleaches clothes, towels, upholstery, and other fabrics. Urge your child to use it with care.

Don't pick. Some kids can't resist the temptation to pick, pop, and squeeze their pimples. Encourage your child to be gentle with his skin. Explain that the pressure caused by squeezing can spread the bacteria, push the infection further into the skin, and increase the risk of permanent scarring.

Know your cosmetics. Some soaps, sunscreens, lotions, and cosmetics can make a bad acne situation worse. Look for products marked "nonacnegenic," meaning they don't cause acne, or those that do not contain oils. Encourage your child to read all cosmetic labels carefully, including the labels on hair-care products, such as gels, mousses, and hair sprays.

Natural Remedies

All of the natural remedies listed below can be used to supplement conventional medical treatment.

Diet and Nutrition

Use one or more of the remedies listed below. Dosage varies according to age; see the chart on pages 14–15 to determine to correct dose for your child. For good food sources of particular nutrients, see pages 9–13.

- Vitamin E (taken internally) reduces scarring and regulates levels of vitamin A in the body. Give your child one dose of vitamin E twice a day for 3 months.
- Zinc improves the condition of the skin and inhibits the conversion of testosterone to DHT, the real acne culprit. Give your child 2–3 doses of zinc a day for 3 months. Be patient, it can sometimes take weeks or even months for the overall condition of the skin to improve.

Herbal

Use one or more of the remedies listed below. Dosage varies according to age; see the chart on page 25 to determine the correct dose for your child.

- Basil kills bacteria on the skin. Prepare an infusion of basil by adding 2 teaspoons of dried basil leaves to 1 cup of boiling water. Allow the leaves to steep for 10–20 minutes. Give your child up to 3 doses of basil tea a day.
- Calendula soap soothes irritated skin and helps fight infection. Have your child wash directly with the herbal soap, making sure to rinse thoroughly with lukewarm water.
- Tea tree oil is considered the ideal skin disinfectant. A solution of 5 percent tea tree oil applied topically, after a thorough cleansing of the area, offers the same benefit as benzoyl peroxide, but has fewer side effects.

Homeopathy

Use one homeopathic treatment at a time, based on your child's specific symptoms. For dosage information, see the chart on pages 31–37. Discontinue use if the symptoms disappear.

- *Calcarea sulph. (Calcarea sulphurica)* 6c: Use for weeping pimples that form yellow crusts. Give 1 dose 3 times daily for up to 2 weeks.
- *Hepar sulph. (Hepar sulphuris calcareum)* 6c: Use for large pimples that look like boils. Give 1 dose 3 times daily for up to 2 weeks.
- *Silicea (Silicea terra)* 6c: Use if the skin scars easily. Give 1 dose 3 times daily for up to 2 weeks.
- *Sulphur* 6c: Use for chronic acne, rough hard skin. Give 1 dose 3 times daily for up to 2 weeks.

Acupressure

Use one or more of the acupressure points listed below. For a diagram showing the specific pressure points, see pages 40–41.

- Four Whites (Stomach 2): This point is located one child's finger width below the lower ridge of the eye socket in line with the center of the iris in an indentation of the cheek.
- Heavenly Pillar (Bladder 10): To find this point, place your fingers ½ inch below the base of the skull on the muscles ½ inch outward from either side of the spine.
- Sea of Vitality (Bladder 23 and Bladder 47): In the lower back, between the second and third lumbar vertebrae, 2–4 child's finger widths away from the spine at waist level.
- Three Mile Point (Stomach 36): This point is located 4 child's finger widths below the kneecap toward the outside of the shinbone.

An Ounce of Prevention

Some children will be acne prone and others will get through adolescence with barely a blemish to show for it. Regardless of predisposition, some acne can be prevented by keeping the skin scrupulously clean, and washing the face twice a day with unscented soap. Encourage your child to avoid oily hair products and makeup. Exposure to a bit of sunlight can also help, but be wary of the damaging effects of the sun. Also note that the chemicals found in some acne medications can cause increased sensitivity to the sun; these products should have a warning on the label.

When to Call for Help

It's hard enough being an adolescent without adding the burden of pimples. If your child tries home remedies for several months to no avail, contact a dermatologist for expert help. Dermatologists can prescribe stronger and more effective drugs that can clear up most cases of adolescent acne. In addition, call a doctor or dermatologist if your child develops a cyst, pustule, or other skin infections that are more than mere pimples.

Allergies

It starts out with a simple sneeze. But when one sneeze turns into three, then five, you suspect the worst: Your child may have allergies.

An allergy is the body's response to an irritant you breathe (such as dust mites, pollen, mold, or pet dander), eat (such as dairy products, wheat, or peanuts), or touch (such as wool, fabric softener, or perfume). Inside the body, this perceived invader or allergen is attacked by IgE antibodies (immunoglobulin E). The antibodies set off a chain reaction that leads to any of a number of symptoms, including runny nose and inflammation of the nasal passages, hives, eczema, arthritis, itching, diarrhea, and headaches.

If the allergies are bad enough, you may want to have your child tested to find out exactly which allergens are causing the problem. Once you know what you're up against, you can try to avoid contact with the substances that bother your child. In the meantime, there are things you can do to steer clear of allergens and to make your child feel better.

Traditional Treatments

Keep a well-stocked medicine cabinet. If your child has allergies, expect to spend a fair amount of time administering medication to deal with the symptoms. Over-the-counter antihistamines help control sneezing, itching, and watery eyes, but they can cause drowsiness. Decongestants can help with a stuffy nose, but won't help a runny nose or sneezing, and they can cause irritability or nervousness. Never give your child over-the-counter nose drops, which may provide temporary relief, but often make the problem worse in the long run.

Kill those mites. Dust mites are one of the most common

allergens, though it's not the mites but their droppings that cause the problem. To minimize mites, consider these suggestions:

- Encase your child's mattress, box spring, and pillow in vinyl, and tape the zippers shut. (Bedding is a favorite nest for dust mites.)
- Give your child washable cotton, foam, or polyester pillows. Say goodbye to feather and down bedding.
- Wash and rinse all clothing and bedding in hot water. Be sure to wash the blankets as well as the sheets at least every 2 weeks.
- Tear out the carpet in your child's bedroom. Replace it with cotton floor rugs, which should be washed every few weeks in hot water.
- To kill mites in the carpeting in the rest of the house, use special allergy control products containing tannic acid. (For proper usage, follow package instructions.) For information on finding the products, see the prevention section at the end of this section.
- Use a damp mop rather than a dry one when dusting floors.
- Replace drapes and venetian blinds with washable curtains or a simple shade.
- Give most of your child's stuffed animals away. Keep only one or two favorites, and wash them regularly.
- Keep the closets clean and well-vacuumed.

Avoid mold to avoid trouble. Many children are allergic to mold, which thrives in households with high humidity. To avoid it:

- Keep the air moving. Run window or ceiling fans, especially in bathrooms and the kitchen.
- Encourage your child to read, but keep books out of your child's bedroom. Mold often grows on books. Store books in another room. Dust them often, and if possible keep them in barrister bookcases or other enclosed areas.
- Clean nonfabric, colorfast surfaces with diluted bleach and other mold-killing cleaners, which kill the bugs in addition to cleaning the grime.

Watch out for pet dander. Your child may love your pet, but the animal's dander (dead skin) may be a big part of the allergy problem. Many people have allergies to cat saliva, which dries on the cat's skin and then becomes airborne. Try to control your child's exposure by doing the following:

- Keep the pets outdoors. At the least, keep the animal out of your child's bedroom.
- Wash your animal once a week. (Most animals hate this, but consider the alternative.)

Avoid pollens. During certain seasons, especially spring and late fall, it's virtually impossible to inhale without getting a nose full of pollen. Still, there are ways to minimize pollen exposure:

- Run the air conditioner, even if it's really nice outside. Turn it on in the car, too.
- Encourage your child to play outside in the middle of the day, rather than early morning or late afternoon when pollen counts are higher.
- Suggest that your child wash his hair when he comes in from playing outside, to get rid of any pollen that might be trapped in the hair.

Natural Remedies

All of the natural remedies listed below can be used to supplement conventional medical treatment.

Diet and Nutrition

Use one or more of the remedies listed below. Dosage varies according to age; see the chart on pages 14–15 to determine to correct dose for your child. For good food sources of particular nutrients, see pages 9–13.

- Beta-carotene is used by the body to make vitamin A; it also soothes irritated mucous membranes associated with allergies. For chronic allergies, give your child one dose of beta-carotene twice a day for 1 month.

- Vitamin C appears to help prevent allergies, as well as asthma. For chronic allergies, give your child one dose of vitamin C 3 times daily for 1 month.

Herbal

Use one or more of the remedies listed below. Dosage varies according to age; see the chart on page 25 to determine the correct dose for your child.

- Ephedra helps fight inflammation associated with allergies and asthma. (In fact, synthetic ephedrine is used in prescription medications specifically for those conditions.) The herb can be very helpful in managing your child's allergies, but it can produce the same potentially dangerous side effects as ephedrine, including: increased blood pressure and heart rate, insomnia, and anxiety. Talk to your doctor before using ephedra in treating your child's allergies.
- Garlic can be helpful in living with allergies that cause a chronic runny nose. Give your child one dose of odorless garlic twice a day for as long as symptoms persist.
- Thyme tea helps relieve congestion. Give your child 1 dose of tea twice daily for up to 2 weeks.

Homeopathy

Use a remedy designed to address your child's specific symptoms. For homeopathic remedies for cough, see page 127; for headaches, see page 181; for runny nose, see page 248; for sore throat, see page 252, and for stuffy nose, see page 265.

Acupressure

Use one or more of the acupressure points listed below. For a diagram showing the specific pressure points, see pages 40–41.

- Bigger Rushing (Liver 3): This point is located on the top of the foot in the valley between the big toe and the second toe.
- Crooked Pond (Large Intestine 11): Apply steady pressure on the point found at the outer edge of the elbow crease.

- Joining the Valley (Large Intestine 4): To find this point, place your fingers on the outside of the child's hand, in the webbing between the thumb and index finger. Find the highest spot of the muscle when the thumb and index fingers are brought closest together.
- Sea of Energy (Conception Vessel 6): Two of your child's finger widths directly below the belly button.

An Ounce of Prevention

The best way to deal with allergies is to avoid exposing your child to the substances that trigger outbreaks. As mentioned, keeping the house scrupulously clean may help prevent allergic reactions. Vacuum cleaners with special dust-trapping filters also may prove beneficial. For more information on vacuums and other products for allergy sufferers, contact:

Allergy Control Products
96 Danbury Road
Ridgefield, CT 06877
(800) 422-DUST

National Allergy Supply
P.O. Box 1658
4400 Georgia Highway 120
Duluth, GA 30136
(800) 522-1448

When to Call for Help

If you suspect your child has allergies, contact your doctor for advice on how to manage your child's specific condition. Allergy medication or allergy shots may be necessary if the condition can't be controlled any other way. Contact the doctor if your child experiences difficulty breathing, or the symptoms of an allergy attack don't clear up within 1 week.

Anemia

Caution: Before self-treatment of anemia, the cause must be diagnosed by a doctor, for an anemia may represent anything from a simple nutrition deficit of iron to a cancer or leukemia.

Most children act like perpetual motion machines, so if your go-go child suddenly becomes perpetually exhausted, you can be sure that something is wrong. If your miniature powerhouse looks pale and acts tired and listless, he may be suffering from iron-deficiency anemia.

In most cases, anemia is a simple problem that is easily treated. Many children don't get enough iron in their diets, especially during growth spurts at 9–18 months, and throughout adolescence. Children need between 6–12 milligrams of iron every day to produce enough red blood cells or hemoglobin to distribute oxygen throughout the body. Without enough red blood cells, your child will feel tired and find it difficult to concentrate, in addition to becoming sick more often than usual. In extreme cases, anemia can cause shortness of breath and overwhelming fatigue.

Iron deficiency is by far the most common cause of anemia, but deficiencies of folic acid, copper, and vitamins B_6 and B_{12} can also interrupt the formation of red blood cells. In fact, there are more than thirty types of anemia, each with its own cause and treatment. If you suspect your child has anemia, contact your doctor for a simple blood test.

Traditional Treatments

Eat up. The most efficient way to boost the iron in your child's bloodstream is to serve more iron-rich foods. Pull a cookbook off the shelf and look for recipes that use liver or red meat. Also, switch to whole-grain breads, which have more iron than most white breads.

Pull out the cast-iron skillet. When you cook acidic foods in cast-iron cookware, trace amounts of iron leach out into the food. Switching to cast-iron skillets provides a painless way to boost the iron content of many foods.

Natural Remedies

All of the natural remedies listed below can be used to supplement conventional medical treatment.

Diet and Nutrition
Use one or more of the remedies listed below.

• Caffeine interferes with the body's ability to absorb iron; eliminate as much caffeine as possible from your child's diet (i.e., cut out the colas). Likewise, pass on the iced tea, which contains tannins that block iron absorption.
• Serve your child foods rich in iron, including: liver, red meat, dried fruit, fortified cereals, dried beans, sausage, fish, eggs, oatmeal, barley, wheat, nuts and seeds, and dark-green leafy vegetables.
• Vitamin C also helps with the absorption of iron. Serve your child foods rich in vitamin C, such as broccoli, green and red peppers, and citrus fruits.

Homeopathy
For dosage information, see the chart on pages 31–37. Discontinue use if the symptoms disappear.

• *Calcarea phos. (Calcarea phosphorica)* 30c: Use for anemia associated with a growth spurt (either in early childhood or adolescence). Give 1 dose twice daily for up to 2 weeks.

An Ounce of Prevention

To prevent anemia, serve your child well-balanced meals, including iron-rich foods. To prevent anemia in infants, breast-feed as long as possible. Breast milk provides your baby with most of the nutrients he needs, including iron.

When to Call for Help

Simple iron-deficiency anemia can be treated at home with changes in diet. However, you should contact your doctor if your child looks pale and seems lethargic and tired; the doctor will perform a simple blood test to rule out other more serious blood disorders. Your pediatrician may also recommend iron supplements.

Animal Bites

Some kids shy away from animals and hesitate to pet even the gentlest among our four-legged friends. Other kids know no fear and recklessly reach out to touch virtually any creature that's covered with fur. Many animals don't want to be touched—at least not without granting their permission—and too often the animal reminds the child of its wishes with a nasty and painful nip or bite.

Animal bites can spread a number of diseases, including rabies, a potentially deadly disease. Rabies can be carried by dogs and cats, but more common carriers are racoons, opossums, skunks, foxes, and bats. Rabid animals look possessed; they may drool or foam at the mouth and attack without provocation.

Human bites can also cause serious infections. Bites from aggressive playmates or siblings that break the skin should be treated the same way as bites from wild animals. Human saliva is replete with potentially dangerous bacteria. Any bite that bleeds should be seen by a doctor, though you can treat superficial nips at home.

Traditional Treatments

It can't be too clean. Your child is going to resist, but you must thoroughly clean the wound site with soap and water, as well as hydrogen peroxide if it is available. After cleaning, soak the injured area for 15–20 minutes in soapy water. Apply a topical antibiotic, and then cover the wound with a bandage or gauze pad.

Just swell. Even nips that don't "break the skin" can damage the delicate skin and cause swelling. Wrap ice (a frozen vegetable package or a can of cold soda) in a clean cloth and hold it against the wound site to reduce swelling. If possible, elevate the injured area above the level of the heart to further reduce swelling.

Don't forget about tetanus. Most parents get so worked up about rabies, they don't think about the risk of tetanus. Bring your child's immunization records with you to the doctor and make sure your child is up-to-date on his tetanus vaccination. Tetanus is part of the series of DTP (Diphtheria, Tetanus, Pertussis) vaccinations that should be administered in several doses between the ages of 2 months and 5 years; a tetanus booster shot is required every 10 years after that time.

Natural Remedies

All of the natural remedies listed below can be used to supplement conventional medical treatment.

Diet and Nutrition

Use one or more of the remedies listed below. Dosage varies according to age; see the chart on pages 14–15 to determine to correct dose for your child. For good food sources of particular nutrients, see pages 9–13.

- Beta-carotene helps heal the skin. Give your child one dose 3 times a day for 1 week.
- Vitamin C helps reduce swelling. Give your child 1 dose 3 times daily for 1 week.

Herbal

Use one or more of the remedies listed below. Dosage varies according to age; see the chart on page 25 to determine the correct dose for your child.

- Garlic helps fight bacterial infections. Give your child one dose of odorless garlic capsules 3 times a day for 4 days.
- Goldenseal is a powerful antibacterial herb. Mix goldenseal powder with enough warm water to form a thick paste. Apply the mixture directly to the wound site after cleaning. Cover with a sterile bandage.
- Tea tree oil helps kill bacteria. Mix 3–4 drops of oil with a half cup of warm water, then pour it over the wound during the cleansing process.

Homeopathy

Use one homeopathic treatment at a time, based on your child's specific symptoms. For dosage information, see the chart on pages 31–37. Discontinue use if the symptoms disappear.

- *Arnica (Arnica montana)* 30c: Use for a wound that is deep or causes a bruise. Give 1 dose every ½ hour for up to 6 doses; then give 1 dose 3 times a day for 3 days.
- *Staphisagria (Delphinium staphisagria)* 6c: Use for a bite that is very painful. Give 1 dose 4 times a day for up to 3 days.

An Ounce of Prevention

More than 1.5 million children are bitten by dogs each year, and thousands of others are attacked by cats and other animals. Some of these animal assaults can be prevented by understanding what to do—and what not to do—when encountering an angry animal. When it comes to dealing with a distraught dog, teach your child these basic tips:

- Never approach an animal you don't know, and never tease or torment any animal.
- Don't run; freeze. A dog will chase you if you run, so you're

better off letting the dog come up to you and sniff you over.
- Don't look directly into the dog's eyes. Staring may be perceived as a challenge to a dog and can prompt an attack.
- Tell him who's boss. Try giving the dog a command such as "sit" or "no." Tell your child to use a firm voice.

When to Call for Help

A bite that breaks the skin by any animal other than your family pet should be seen by a doctor. Bites by dogs or cats whose owners can't show proof of immunization require that the animal be observed for 10 days to 2 weeks for signs of sickness or rabies. With wild animals, stray dogs or cats, or animals that show signs of illness, your child may have to undergo a series of injections to prevent rabies. In addition, a tetanus booster may be required if your child's vaccinations have not been kept up to date.

Animal bites also present a threat of infection, caused by bacteria living in the animal's mouth. Clean all wound sites meticulously and contact your doctor at the first signs of infection, including: fever, redness and swelling of the wound site, and pus or discharge from the wound itself.

Asthma

Nine out of ten cases of childhood asthma are triggered by allergies. When the child inhales the allergen, the muscles in the bronchial tubes spasm and mucus builds up, making it difficult to breathe. Then airways begin to swell, further narrowing the breathing passages.

During an asthma attack, your child might cough, wheeze, and complain of tightness in the chest. Some attacks are mild, others may be life-threatening. Asthma can be triggered by a number of irritants, including: pollen, dust, mold, animal dander, air pollution, and viral or bacterial infections. Even exercise can bring on an attack.

Asthma should be treated and monitored by a doctor. Your child may be given medication to prevent attacks, as well as a bronchodilator to open restricted airways during attacks. You should try to identify the allergens that trigger attacks in your child so that you can avoid them.

Traditional Treatments

The best defense . . . is a clean house. Take pains to "allergy-proof" your house by eliminating as many potential sources of allergens as possible. Cover your child's mattress with plastic; remove the carpet from your child's bedroom, and vacuum all rugs frequently. Keep your house—and especially your child's bedroom—as clean and free of dust and mold as possible. (For more information on dealing with allergies, see page 58.)

Know the flow. Your child's doctor may give your child a device known as a peak-flow meter, which measures how much air makes its way to the lungs. Have your child use the device first thing every morning; you may be able to recognize problem days and adjust the levels of medication to avoid dangerous asthma attacks. Keep a diary of your child's meter readings, attacks, and medications to try to distinguish patterns and tip-offs of when attacks will occur.

Develop a game plan. Start by holding a meeting with everyone involved with your child's care, including teachers or day-care supervisors. Explain the condition and go over exactly what procedures should be followed if your child has an asthma attack. Older children may use metered-dose inhalers to take their medication, and you should practice with your child how to use the devices properly (they can be tricky). Also practice staying calm; the more nervous you are, the more nervous your child will be.

Always have a backup. When your child has an asthma attack, you need to have the medicine—now. As a precaution, always keep at least one extra, full metered-dose inhaler on hand. Try to keep one on every floor of your house. (Don't leave one in the car, however, since extreme heat can cause the canisters to leak or explode.) When you buy a new inhaler, use the backup and replace it with the new medicine so that the extra inhaler does not get old and out of date. (Most inhalers are good for about 2 years, but you should always check the expiration date on the product.)

Go ahead and let him exercise. Asthma should not prevent your child from being active, though it may require that you give him a prophylactic dose of medication before a workout or athletic event. Talk to your child's pediatrician to determine the correct dosage.

Natural Remedies

All of the natural remedies listed below can be used to supplement conventional medical treatment.

Diet and Nutrition

Use one or more of the remedies listed below. Dosage varies according to age; see the chart on pages 14–15 to determine to correct dose for your child. For good food sources of particular nutrients, see pages 9–13.

- Vitamin B_6 supplementation has been shown to be beneficial to children with asthma. Talk to your child's doctor about an appropriate vitamin regimen, since extremely high doses of vitamin B_6 can be toxic.
- Vitamin C helps reduce the number and intensity of asthma attacks, since it acts in the body as an anti-inflammatory. Give your child 1 dose of vitamin C 3 times a day for 1 month, and look for a change in frequency and severity of attacks.

Herbal

Dosage varies according to age; see the chart on page 25 to determine the correct dose for your child.

- Evening primrose oil helps regulate inflammation and, therefore, helps alleviate asthma. Give your child 1 dose twice daily for 2 months, following the product dosage guidelines.

Homeopathy

Use one homeopathic treatment at a time, based on your child's specific symptoms. For dosage information, see the chart on pages 31–37. Discontinue use if the symptoms disappear.

- *Aconite (Aconitum napellus)* 30c: Use if an asthma attack comes on suddenly, especially after exposure to cold, dry wind. Give 1 dose every 10 minutes for up to 10 doses.
- *Arsenicum (Arsenicum album)* 6c: Use if an attack comes at night. Give 1 dose every 10 minutes for up to 10 doses.
- *Carbo veg. (Carbo vegetabilis)* 30c: Use if the attack involves coughing, gagging, and fighting for air. Give 1 dose every 10 minutes for up to 10 doses.
- *Kali carb. (Kali carbonicum)* 6c: Use if an asthma attack strikes in the early morning (around 4 A.M.). Give 1 dose every 10 minutes for up to 10 doses.

Acupressure

Use one or more of the acupressure points listed below. For a diagram showing the specific pressure points, see pages 40–41.

- Great Abyss (Lung 9): This point is located in the groove at the wrist fold below the base of the thumb.
- Letting Go (Lung 1): To find this point, place your fingers on the outer part of the chest, 3 child's finger widths below the collarbone.
- Lung Associated Point (Bladder 13): Apply steady pressure on the point 1 child's finger width below the upper tip of the shoulder blade, between the spine and the scapula.

An Ounce of Prevention

To avoid asthma attacks, your child must avoid the allergens or activities that trigger the attacks. If your child's asthma stems from exercise rather than allergies, talk to your doctor about administering a preventive dose of asthma medication before your child engages in any physical activity.

When to Call for Help

Asthma should always be treated and monitored by a physician, preferably one with experience treating asthmatics. It's often hard to know when to call for help—but if you're in doubt, err on the side of caution and call the doctor—and you should always seek medical help if your child is fighting for breath and cannot talk, is sitting still and leaning forward to try to get air, or does not improve within 10 minutes of taking the medication. Asthma is a life-threatening condition, and every attack should be treated with respect.

Athlete's Foot

Athlete's foot doesn't discriminate: It afflicts both couch potatoes and toned jocks with equal vigor. Athlete's foot (*tinea pedis*) is actually a fungal infection caused by the same fungus that causes jock itch and ringworm. It earned its name because the fungus thrives in the damp, moist environment typical of most locker-room floors.

The athlete's foot fungus causes itching, burning, scaling, cracking, and stinging feet. It is rare in children under 10, but common in adolescence and adulthood. The fungus is highly contagious, but for unknown reasons, it does seem to be more prevalent in certain unfortunate, predisposed individuals.

Traditional Treatments

- *No sweat.* To get rid of the fungus, your child is going to have to keep his feet clean and dry. Make sure your child takes a few minutes after showering or bathing to carefully dry between his toes. A blast with a hair dryer between the toes might help eliminate any remaining moisture. When weather permits, have your child wear sandals or light shoes to let as much air as possible reach his feet, to allow for evaporation of sweat.

- *Change is good.* Shoes need a chance to dry out between wearings; have your child alternate between two or more pairs of shoes or sneakers.
- *Dust 'em off.* You can cut down on moisture in your child's shoes by dusting his feet and the inside of the shoes with an over-the-counter antifungal powder. A number of products are available at pharmacies. You may notice results in as little as 3–4 days, or it may take 3–4 weeks, depending on the tenacity of the fungus.
- *Bring back the happy feet.* Soothe the sores by soaking your child's cracked or oozing feet in a bath made with Burow's Solution or Domeboro powder, antiseptic products sold over-the-counter. Follow package directions.

Natural Remedies

All of the natural remedies listed below can be used to supplement conventional medical treatment.

Diet and Nutrition

Use one or more of the remedies listed below. Dosage varies according to age; see the chart on pages 14–15 to determine to correct dose for your child. For good food sources of particular nutrients, see pages 9–13.

- Lactobacillus acidophilus supplements encourage the growth of "good" bacteria that help fight fungal infections. Follow package directions for appropriate dosage.
- Cut sweets out of your child's diet since sugar encourages growth of the fungus.
- Zinc helps heal skin tissue. Give your child 1 dose per day for 1–2 weeks.

Herbal

Use one or more of the remedies listed below. Dosage varies according to age; see the chart on page 25 to determine the correct dose for your child.

- The athlete's foot fungus will not thrive in an acidic environment. Soak your child's feet in apple cider vinegar (diluted 1 part vinegar to 4 parts water) or wipe between the toes with a washcloth soaked in undiluted vinegar.
- Aloe vera gel and calendula ointment can be used on alternate days to soothe and heal red, itchy skin.
- Garlic is excellent at fighting infection. Give your child 2 or 3 doses of odorless garlic capsules a day, or dust the affected feet and toes with garlic powder.
- Tea tree oil is an excellent antifungal herbal treatment. Twice a day, soak your child's feet for 10 minutes in a soothing foot bath consisting of one quart of warm water and 10–15 drops of tea tree oil. Dry the feet thoroughly, especially between the toes, then apply undiluted tea tree oil directly to the affected areas and leave on the skin.

Homeopathy

For dosage information, see the chart on pages 31–37. Discontinue use if the symptoms disappear.

- *Thuja (Thuja occidentalis)* (undiluted): Rub directly on the affected areas twice a day.

An Ounce of Prevention

If your child is susceptible to athlete's foot, take strides to keep his feet as clean and dry as possible. Have him wear white cotton socks that allow feet to breathe, and wash the socks in chlorine bleach after each wearing to kill any fungus that might be present.

Some kids have sweaty feet that provide a prime breeding ground for fungus. If your child has wet feet, have him change his socks 2 or 3 times a day to keep his feet as dry as possible. In addition, when weather permits, have him wear sandals or open shoes to allow air to reach the feet. And, of course, have your child wear waterproof slippers or sandals in locker rooms and public showers to avoid direct contact with the fungus.

When to Call for Help

Athlete's foot can usually be defeated by consistent and aggressive home treatment. The fungal infection can be accompanied by a bacterial infection, however, which could require medical attention. If the condition persists—or gets worse—after about a month of do-it-yourself care, call a doctor.

Bad Breath

Often, bad breath (*halitosis*) has less to do with what you eat than how well you clean your teeth after you've finished eating. That's why children, most of whom refuse to nosh on garlic, onions, blue cheese, and other strong-smelling foods, can fall prey to bad breath just as often as adults do.

Bad breath is usually caused by a buildup of bacteria in the mouth. Morning breath often smells particularly fragrant because the mouth tends to dry out overnight, giving bacteria a chance to flourish, even in your sweet little two-year-old's mouth.

Traditional Treatments

- *Brush, brush, brush.* Brushing the teeth properly is the first line of defense against bad breath. Assist your child, if necessary, making sure your child spends enough time carefully scrubbing each tooth. This oral hygiene routine should take at least 3–5 minutes; wetting the toothbrush and smearing toothpaste in the mouth isn't going to remove all the tiny food particles trapped between the teeth. Older kids with braces or other orthodontic devices need to spend even more time cleaning in, around, and between the hardware.

- *Floss, floss, floss.* Older children should add flossing to their tooth-care routine once they're capable of gently and thoroughly managing the chore. Talk to your dentist about when to add flossing to your child's dental regimen.

- *Make brushing fun.* Some kids enjoy the thrill of high-tech brushing, so using an electric toothbrush or fancy rotary-cleaning model can be a good way of getting your child to brush properly. These devices often do a good job of cleaning the teeth, and your child is more likely to brush longer and more often if he enjoys the process.

- *Don't stop with the teeth.* Though it may tickle a bit at first, have your child gently brush his tongue to remove plaque-causing bacteria from the mouth. Some studies show that brushing the tongue fights foul-smelling breath better than brushing the teeth. This is one time when you'll want to encourage your child to stick out his tongue—for a good brushing.

- *Dry mouth, smelly mouth.* If your child has a problem with cotton mouth, especially when he feels anxious or stressed, encourage him to drink plenty of water to keep his mouth moist and well lubricated. Saliva helps rinse food particles and debris away, preventing bad breath. Offering your child sugarless candies or chewing gum can stimulate saliva flow, but steer clear of products containing sugar, since bacteria that cause bad breath thrive on sweets.

- *Don't wash your mouth out.* At least not with mouthwash. Children under age 6 should skip fluoride mouthwash rinses because they often swallow the fluid, which usually contains significant quantities of alcohol. Older children can use the products, but you may want to dilute them with 1 or 2 parts water to 1 part mouthwash.

Natural Remedies

All of the natural remedies listed below can be used to supplement conventional medical treatment.

Diet and Nutrition
Use one or more of the remedies listed below. Dosage varies according to age; see the chart on pages 14–15 to determine to correct dose for your child. For good food sources of particular nutrients, see pages 9–13.

- Chlorophyll tablets freshen the breath. In fact, chlorophyll is the active ingredient in many commercial breath mints. For proper use, follow dosage directions on the product label.
- Eating citrus fruits can stimulate the production of saliva and freshen breath. When bad breath is a problem, encourage your child to snack on a tangy orange, grapefruit, or other citrus fruit.
- Lactobacillus acidophilus helps maintain healthy intestinal bacteria, which can improve bad breath caused by digestive problems. Give your child one dose of the supplement daily; see dosage information on the product label for effective use.

Herbal

- That parsley on your plate isn't just there for show. Parsley freshens breath because it contains high levels of chlorophyll. Encourage your child to eat his parsley to remedy bad breath.

Homeopathy
Use one homeopathic treatment at a time, based on your child's specific symptoms. For dosage information, see the chart on pages 31–37. Discontinue use if the symptoms disappear.

- *Aurum (Aurum metallicum)* 6c: Use as often as necessary if your child experiences bad breath during the onset of puberty. Give 3 times daily for up to 5 days.

- *Nux (Strychnos nux vomica)* 6c: Use if your child's breath smells sour after an upset stomach. Give 3 times daily for up to 5 days.
- *Pulsatilla (Pulsatilla nigricans)* 6c: Use if your child has bad breath after eating fatty foods. Give 3 times daily for up to 5 days.

An Ounce of Prevention

Most bad breath can be prevented by practicing good oral hygiene. Be sure your child visits the dentist for checkups every 6 months. If possible, encourage your child to carry a toothbrush, and to use it after meals and snacks. If brushing isn't realistic, have your child rinse his mouth with water after eating and encourage him to snack on raw vegetables, which are not only good for him but also help clean the teeth.

When to Call for Help

Bad breath can usually be cured with a few simple home remedies, but chronic foul breath in children demands medical attention. If a yellow nasal discharge accompanies the odor, contact your doctor. Sometimes toddlers shove small objects up their noses, which become blocked and infected, causing bad breath.

Less-than-sweet breath can also be caused by other illnesses that result in mouth-breathing, such as an infection of the sinuses, tonsils, or adenoids, or something as simple as allergies or a stuffy nose. Call a medical professional if your child experiences fever, diarrhea, or abdominal cramping in addition to bad breath. Of course, dental problems often show up as bad breath, so contact a dentist if your child has obvious signs of dental decay, loose teeth, or bleeding gums.

Bed-Wetting

It's hard for a child with a bed-wetting problem to greet the morning with anything other than anxiety and shame. Most of the time, bed-wetting is caused by a small bladder, which simply cannot physically hold urine through the night. Bladder size is often hereditary: If you wet the bed as a child, there's a 1 in 2 chance that your child will, too; if both you and your spouse were bed-wetters, the odds jump to 3 out of 4.

Bed-wetting (*enuresis*) isn't considered a problem until your child is at least 5 or 6 years old. And even at that age, almost 1 out of 5 kids (a disproportionate number of them boys) can't "hold it" all night. Unless there is an underlying physical problem, kids with tiny bladders will eventually outgrow the problem.

But in the meantime, bed-wetting can be torture on a kid, making summer camp and sleepovers an embarrassing prospect. You can help your child manage his bed-wetting and deal with occasional accidents during high stress periods (such as when starting school or welcoming a new baby) by following a few basic tips.

Traditional Treatments

It's not such a big deal. Bed-wetting can be humiliating to a child, so be sensitive to his embarrassment. Explain to your child that his bladder isn't big enough yet, and that you can help him deal with the problem. Don't punish or tease your child. Instead, buy a plastic mattress cover, show your child where the clean sheets are stored, and help him manage the problem on his own. (Of course, you can lend a hand with

79

making the bed, but the more responsibility left to the child, the better.)

Don't wake him up. Bed-wetting is your child's problem, not yours. Don't wake your child up in the night to take him to the bathroom or you will teach your child that bladder control is your responsibility, not his.

Congratulations! Acknowledge dry nights, perhaps even by giving your child a sticker as a reward, in addition to kind words and a pat on the back. Ignore wet mornings altogether.

Practice makes perfect. During the day, help your child "train" his bladder to hold more urine. Ask your child to drink several glasses of water and wait as long as he can to urinate. Then, when he can't hold on any longer, have him try to stop urinating midstream to work on control of the bladder sphincter. These exercises will stretch the bladder and teach your child how to manage the feeling associated with a full bladder. Of course, encourage your child to cut back on fluids after dinnertime so he won't head to bed with a full bladder.

You have my permission. Some kids won't leave their beds at night because they're afraid of the dark or afraid to violate the order to stay in bed. Explain to your child that he can get out of bed to use the toilet. If necessary, plug in a night-light or give your child a flashlight to make wandering to the bathroom feel less frightening.

Go to bed earlier. Some kids wet the bed because they're just too exhausted to heed their body's natural urges in the night. If your child is wetting the bed, he may be sleeping so soundly that he can't wake up when his bladder needs to be emptied. Try an earlier bedtime and see if the situation improves.

Is the bed talking to you? Some kids respond well to bed alarms, which either sound a warning or vibrate at the first sign of moisture hitting the bed. These battery-operated pads cost about $45, and help the child associate the physical sensation of urination with the bladder pressure they feel at night. Bed alarms should only be used if your child *wants* to try them out.

Natural Remedies

All of the natural remedies listed below can be used to supplement conventional medical treatment.

Diet and Nutrition

- Caffeine is a diuretic; it encourages urination. Avoid caffeine in your child's diet, especially after dinner.

Homeopathy

Use one homeopathic treatment at a time, based on your child's specific symptoms. For dosage information, see the chart on pages 31–37. Discontinue use if the symptoms disappear.

- *Calcarea phos. (Calcarea phosphorica)* 30x or 9c: Use if your child urinates only a small amount during the night without awakening. Give 1 dose twice a day (in the morning and before bed) for up to 2 weeks.
- *Causticum (Causticum hahnemanni)* 30x or 9c: Use if you check on your child before you go to sleep and find that he has wet the bed early in the night. Give 1 dose twice a day (in the morning and before bed) for up to 2 weeks.
- *Equisetum (Equisetum byemale)* 30x or 9c: Use if your child soaks the bed and complains of abdominal pain. Give 1 dose twice a day (in the morning and before bed) for up to 2 weeks.

Acupressure

Use one or more of the acupressure points listed below. For a diagram showing the specific pressure points, see pages 40–41.

- Bigger Stream (Kidney 3): To find this point, place your fingers in the hollow midway between the protrusion of the inside anklebone and the Achilles tendon, which joins the back of the calf to the back of the heel.
- Gate Origin (Conception Vessel 4): This point is located 4 child's finger widths below the belly button.

An Ounce of Prevention

Most cases of bed-wetting occur because your child's bladder simply isn't large enough to accommodate a full night's worth of urine. In such cases, the only solution to the bed-wetting problem is time, so be patient with your child. While you're waiting for nature to take its course, allow your child to use diapers at night, until he's awakened "dry" on 3 or 4 nights in a row. Also, avoid drinking fluids at night and steer clear of caffeine.

When to Call for Help

Most of the time, bed-wetting is a harmless (if unpleasant) problem for a child. However, a lack of bladder control can indicate physical problems, such as urinary tract infections or diabetes. Call the pediatrician if your child complains of pain during urination, frequent thirst, or abdominal and/or back pain. Also contact the doctor if your child wets during the day as well as at night, develops a bed-wetting problem after a prolonged period of dryness, or wets frequently even though he is more than 5 years old.

Black Eyes

Black eyes: Some kids wear them like a badge of honor, while others shrink away from all the fuss and attention they stir up. Whether caused by a missed fly ball in the outfield or an unfortunate run-in with the class bully on the playground, black eyes are the body's way of announcing to the world that your child has suffered a bump or bruise to the head.

Black eyes look more dramatic than bruises elsewhere on the body because the area surrounding the eye is replete with tiny blood vessels and the skin is thinner and more sensitive in that area. After the injury, blood leaks from this network of vessels into the surrounding tissue and a few hours later your child has a real shiner.

Fortunately, the blood vessels in the face usually heal quickly. The red, purple, and black bruises will gradually change color and fade as the body reabsorbs the blood.

Traditional Treatments

- *Ice is nice.* In years past, the common remedy for a black eye was a nice, cold steak compress. This remedy worked, not because the red meat had any medicinal value, but because the cool meat kept the swelling down by constricting the blood vessels. An ice pack, a can of cool soda, or a bag of frozen vegetables will work just as well (and cost much less). No matter what you use, put the compress against the cheek and around the eye, not over the eyeball itself, and wrap the frozen item in a cloth or rag to prevent frostbite. Put the ice on the bruise for 5–10 minutes, then remove it for 15–20 minutes. Repeat this cycle for several hours after the injury, and as often as your child will tolerate it for the next day or so.
- *Warmth for healing.* Two days after the injury, apply a warm compress (using the same on-again, off-again timing). This will help the mark fade by encouraging the body to reabsorb the pooled blood.
- *Ease the pain.* If your child has either a headache or general achiness, give him some acetaminophen to ease the pain. Check the package directions for the correct dosage. Don't use ibuprofen, since it can increase bleeding because of its anticlotting properties. And, of course, never give a child under age 18 aspirin (even ''baby aspirin'') for any reason, because it has been linked to Reye's syndrome, a potentially life-threatening disorder.

Natural Remedies

All of the natural remedies listed below can be used to supplement conventional medical treatment.

Diet and Nutrition

Dosage varies according to age; see the chart on pages 14–15 to determine to correct dose for your child. For good food sources of particular nutrients, see pages 9–13.

- To help heal the walls of the blood vessels, give your child a ½ dose of vitamin C 3 times a day for a week. In addition, encourage your child to eat pineapple and papaya, which contain enzymes that help the body absorb the blood that causes the bruising.

Homeopathy

Use one homeopathic treatment at a time, based on your child's specific symptoms. For dosage information, see the chart on pages 31–37. Discontinue use if the symptoms disappear.

- *Arnica (Arnica montana)* 30x or 9c: Use if the black eye follows a blow to head or eyes. Give immediately after the injury, and every 4 hours after for up to 10 doses.
- *Ledum (Ledum palustre)* 12x or 6c: Use if the discoloration persists, or if the pain is relieved by applying a cold compress. Give every 4 hours for up to 10 doses.

Acupressure

Use one or more of the acupressure points listed below. For a diagram showing the specific pressure points, see pages 40–41.

- Joining the Valley (Large Intestine 4): This point is located in the webbing between the thumb and index finger at the highest spot of the muscle where the thumb and index finger are closest together.
- Sea of Vitality (Bladder 23 and Bladder 47): In the lower back, between the second and third lumbar vertebrae, 2–4 finger widths away from the spine at waist level.

An Ounce of Prevention

Try as you may, you can't stop your children from experiencing the common bumps and bruises of childhood. Do your best to minimize accidents; then, when the inevitable occurs, be ready to comfort your child with a hug, a kiss, and appropriate medical care.

When to Call for Help

A black eye is serious business. As a matter of course, have your doctor take a look at your child's injury if he develops a black eye to rule out the possibility of concussion or injury to the eye. After all, if your child was clobbered hard enough to cause a black-and-blue mark on his face, then the impact was certainly significant enough to potentially damage the delicate tissues of the eye.

Contact your doctor or an ophthalmologist again if your child experiences eye pain, blurred or double vision, the perception of something "floating" in the field of vision, light sensitivity, or other vision irregularities. Also, keep an eye out for irregularly shaped or clouded pupils, discharge from the eye, or increasing redness. If your child develops two black eyes following a blow to the head, call for emergency assistance; the bruises may indicate a fracture at the base of the skull.

Boils

You might tell your kids not to make mountains out of molehills, but when your child develops a boil, you can be sure that the red, swollen bump feels like Mount McKinley. A boil forms when the bacterium *staphylococcus aureau* invades the body through a hair follicle or a cut in the skin. Under the skin, the staph bacteria multiply, then the body's infection-fighting mechanism kicks in and floods the area with white blood cells, forming pus. The painful result: A tender, red mound that may hang around for two or three weeks before either coming to a head and bursting or gradually fading away.

Boils can erupt anywhere on the body, but they often appear on the neck, face, buttocks, and underarms. Children fall prey to boils more often than adults because they are more apt to suffer scrapes and scratches and encounter staph bacteria when playing outdoors. While boils can be painful and unsightly, they respond well to home treatment and natural remedies.

Traditional Treatment

- *Bring it to a head.* Apply warm compresses on the boil for 10 or 15 minutes, 4 or more times a day. The heat and moisture will help draw the pus and infection up to the surface of the skin, where it can drain.
- *Please, don't squeeze.* Pinching, popping, and poking the boil can spread the infection under the skin and cause scarring. More importantly, squeezing some boils—particularly those near the lips, nose, in the armpits, and the groin—can force the infection into the bloodstream, where it can cause blood poisoning.

Natural Remedies

All of the natural remedies listed below can be used to supplement conventional medical treatment.

Diet and Nutrition

Use one or more of the remedies listed below. Dosage varies according to age; see the chart on pages 14–15 to determine to correct dose for your child. Some vitamins can be used topically, as noted. For good food sources of particular nutrients, see pages 9–13.

- If the boil has not come to a head, open a vitamin A capsule directly onto the boil, twice a day, for up to 5 days, to help it heal.
- Apply a few drops of vitamin E directly to the boil after it has come to a head to help minimize scarring.
- Zinc helps heal the skin and boost the immune system. Give your child one dose of zinc, twice a day, for 1 week, or until healed.

Herbal
Use one or more of the remedies listed below. Dosage varies according to age; see the chart on page 25 to determine the correct dose for your child.

- Prepare a strong ginger tea and make a compress with it by soaking a clean cloth in the mixture, and applying it to the boil for 15 minutes, 4 times a day. The ginger tea will help bring the boil to a head and draw out the infection.
- Steep 1 tablespoon of goldenseal and ½ teaspoon of myrrh in a pint of boiling water, and use to wash the infected area.
- Try a compress of tea tree oil, a strong antiseptic that can help clear up the infection. Add 8–10 drops of tea tree oil to 1 quart of hot water. Soak a clean cloth in the mixture and apply to the boil for 15 minutes, 4 times a day.

Homeopathy
Use one homeopathic treatment at a time, based on your child's specific symptoms. For dosage information, see the chart on pages 31–37. Discontinue use if the symptoms disappear.

- *Belladonna (Atropa belladonna)* 30x or 9c: Use when the boil first appears. Give 1 dose every 4 hours for 1 day.
- *Hepar sulph. (Hepar sulphuris calcareum)* 12x or 6c: Use when a head appears on the boil, or if it is very sensitive to touch. Give 1 dose 3 times daily for 1 day.
- *Myristica (Myristica sebifera)* 12x or 6c: Use to promote draining of the pus. Give 1 dose 4 times daily for 1 day.
- *Silicea (Silicea terra)* 6c: Use to cleanse and heal a boil that has already drained. Give 1 dose 4 times daily for 1 day.

An Ounce of Prevention

Boils happen, particularly in hot, humid conditions. Some unfortunate souls are born into families cursed with a propensity toward developing boils, but most people can minimize their chances of developing them by keeping their skin clean and dry. If your child is prone to boils, consider using an antiseptic soap to kill staph bacteria. Check your child's skin after a few days to make sure it isn't dry and irritated; some people find antiseptic soaps too astringent to use on a regular basis. If your child's skin is too delicate to handle strong soaps, try using the antiseptic soap every other day.

To prevent the spread of boils to other parts of the body, have your child take showers instead of baths when the boil is draining. Likewise, be sure your child thoroughly washes his hands before eating, since the same staph bacteria also may cause food poisoning.

When to Call for Help

Boils deserve your care and attention, and they demand medical attention if there are signs that the infection has spread. Call your doctor if your child has a fever or swollen lymph nodes, if red streaks appear around the boil, or if it stubbornly refuses to disappear after several weeks of home treatment. Also contact your doctor if your child develops a boil on the face, especially around the mouth and nose, since there is a possibility that the bacteria can spread to the blood or sinuses.

Your doctor may lance or make a small cut in the center of the boil to drain the pus. After draining, many physicians prescribe an antibiotic to keep the infection from coming back. After lancing, you can use natural remedies to prevent scarring, just as you would if it drained on its own.

Bronchitis

Just when you think the end is in sight, the coughing begins. At first, your child seems to be getting better: The cold and flu symptoms subside, but then your little one comes up with a hacking cough and sudden fever. Time for a round of bronchitis.

Bronchitis is an inflammation of the windpipe and the large bronchial tubes that branch off into the lungs. It can be triggered by a bacterial or viral infection or by an allergic reaction to something your child has inhaled, such as pollens, cat dander, or dust. As the lining of the bronchi swell, mucus builds up, causing an irresistible urge to cough and clear the throat.

Most bouts with bronchitis last only a week or so. If symptoms persist, call your doctor, who can determine if the condition is caused by a bacterial infection, in which case antibiotics may be needed. Regardless of the cause of the bronchitis, there are a number of things you can do to make your child more comfortable while waiting for the condition to clear.

Traditional Treatments

How about another glass? Give your child as much water or other fluids as he will drink. The liquids thin the mucus in the lungs, making it easier for your child to cough it up.

Keep it misty and moist. Keep the humidifier or vaporizer running on "high" in your child's bedroom throughout the night, to elevate the humidity in the room. The moisture keeps the lungs moist and reduces the irritation and scratchy feeling in your child's throat.

Consider drugs. Over-the-counter *expectorants* help loosen the mucus to make coughing more productive; these products are most helpful during the day. Over-the-counter cough *suppressants* for children can be used at night to help your child get a good night's sleep, but should not be used during the day since coughing is necessary to clear the mucus out of the lungs.

Soup's on. Chicken soup will not only make your child feel nurtured and loved, it will also help clear away the congestion. Grandma was right: Chicken soup really does do a better job than other hot liquids at opening blocked breathing passages. Homemade is a special treat, but store-bought works just as well.

Natural Remedies

All of the natural remedies listed below can be used to supplement conventional medical treatment.

Diet and Nutrition
Use one or more of the remedies listed below. Dosage varies according to age; see the chart on pages 14–15 to determine to correct dose for your child. For good food sources of particular nutrients, see pages 9–13.

- Beta-carotene helps clear bronchitis, and soothe the mucous membranes. Give your child 1 dose twice daily for 3–4 days.
- Vitamin C helps reduce inflammation. Give your child 1 dose 3 times a day for up to 1 week.

Herbal
Dosage varies according to age; see the chart on page 25 to determine the correct dose for your child.

- Thyme helps kill microbes and reduce coughing. Give your child 1 dose of thyme tea 3 times a day for 3–4 days.

Homeopathy
Use one homeopathic treatment at a time, based on your child's specific symptoms. For dosage information, see the chart on pages 31–37. Discontinue use if the symptoms disappear.

- *Bryonia (Bryonia alba)* 30c: Use if your child has a painful cough that is worse at night, and if there is chest pain. Give 1 dose 3 times a day for up to 3 days.
- *Ipecac. (Cephaelis ipecacuanha)* 6c: Use if your child has nausea, vomiting, and a suffocating feeling in the chest. Give 1 dose 3 times a day, for up to 3 days.
- *Kali bichrom. (Kali bichromicum)* 12x or 6c: Use if your child has a cough with thick, stringy mucus. Give 1 dose 3 times a day, for up to 3 days.
- *Pulsatilla (Pulsatilla nigricans)* 30x or 9c: Use if your child has a cough accompanied by a runny nose and thin, yellow mucus. Give 1 dose 3 times a day, for up to 3 days.

Acupressure

Use one or more of the acupressure points listed below. For a diagram showing the specific pressure points, see pages 40–41.

- Heaven Rushing Out (Conception Vessel 22): This point is located at the base of the throat, in the large hollow directly below the Adam's apple.
- Letting Go (Lung 1): To find this point, place your fingers on the outer part of the upper chest, 4 child's finger widths up from the armpit crease and 1 finger width inward.
- Vital Diaphragm (Bladder 38): Apply steady pressure on the point between the shoulder blade and the spine at the level of the heart.

An Ounce of Prevention

You can't prevent every cold, but you may be able to prevent some colds from turning into bronchitis by treating them as soon as the first symptoms develop. If your child has allergies, take steps to minimize respiratory problems by avoiding exposure to allergens.

When to Call for Help

Most cases of bronchitis can be treated at home and run their course in 10 days or so. However, call your doctor if you suspect that an infant has bronchitis, or if your child experiences a fever of 103 degrees or higher, extreme lethargy, wheezing, or difficulty breathing. With small children, the airways can swell shut, so seek immediate medical attention if you suspect the problem is growing worse.

Bruises

Bruises are an inevitable part of learning to walk and jump and ride a bike. Your child is going to experience bumps and falls—and the black-and-blue marks that follow—even if you watch with unfailing diligence.

Bruises happen beneath the skin. The classic purplish-red marks appear when an injury to a blood vessel causes blood to leak into the surrounding tissue. These marks, known as hematomas, usually heal within a week or so, often changing from blue to red to yellow to green as they heal.

Traditional Treatments

- *Get a leg up.* Or an arm, if that's where the bruise is located. You want to raise the injured limb above the level of your child's heart to reduce the blood flow and swelling.
- *Keep cool.* After elevating the limb, apply an ice pack, cold soda can, or bag of frozen vegetables to the affected area. Wrap the frozen item in a cloth or rag and avoid direct contact with the skin to prevent frostbite. Put the ice on the bruise for 5–10 minutes, then remove it for 15–20 minutes. Repeat this cycle for several hours after the injury, and as often as your child will tolerate it for the next day or so. The cold will constrict the blood vessels and minimize blood

flow, and it will also prevent the nerves from sending pain messages to the brain.

- *Running hot and cold.* When the classic black-and-blue mark appears, it's time to switch from cold compresses to hot compresses, or a hot water bottle or heating pad. You should use the same timing technique as with the warm treatments, which will promote healing by dilating blood vessels and bringing fresh blood to the site.
- *Don't make matters worse.* If your child complains of a headache or general discomfort, you can give him acetaminophen, following the package directions for the correct dosage. Don't use aspirin or ibuprofen because both drugs can increase bleeding due to their anticlotting properties. For children under 18, aspirin also has been linked to Reye's syndrome, a potentially life-threatening disorder.

Natural Remedies

All of the natural remedies listed below can be used to supplement conventional medical treatment.

Diet and Nutrition
Dosage varies according to age; see the chart on pages 14–15 to determine to correct dose for your child. For good food sources of particular nutrients, see pages 9–13.

- To help heal the walls of the blood vessels, give your child a ½ dose of vitamin C 3 times a day for a week. In addition, encourage your child to eat pineapple and papaya, which contain enzymes that helps the body absorb the blood that causes bruising.

Homeopathy
Use one homeopathic treatment at a time, based on your child's specific symptoms. For dosage information, see the chart on pages 31–37. Discontinue use if the symptoms disappear.

- *Arnica (Arnica montana)* 30x or 9c: Use for bruises caused by an injury. Give 1 dose immediately after the injury, and then 3 times daily, for up to 10 doses.

- *Ledum (Ledum palustre)* 12x or 6c: Use if the discoloration persists, or if the pain is relieved by applying a cold compress. Give 1 dose every 4 hours, for up to 10 doses.
- *Ruta (Ruta graveolens)* 6c: Use if bruises feel as if they are on the bone. Give 1 dose every 8 hours, for up to 10 doses.

Acupressure

Use one or more of the acupressure points listed below. For a diagram showing the specific pressure points, see pages 40–41.

- **Heavenly Appearance (Small Intestine 17):** This point is located in the indentation directly below the earlobe and behind the jawbone.
- **Sea of Vitality (Bladder 23 and Bladder 47):** To find this point, place your fingers between the second and third lumbar vertebrae in the lower back, 2–4 child's finger widths away from the spine at waist level.
- **Three Mile Point (Stomach 36):** Apply steady pressure on the point 4 child's finger widths below the kneecap toward the outside of the shinbone.

An Ounce of Prevention

Kids bruise easily—and often. Of course, you should do what you can to anticipate and avoid accidents, but they will happen despite your efforts. The best you can do is to stand ready to comfort and care for your child—and keep the ice packs ready.

When to Call for Help

Bruises are an everyday part of childhood. However, some bruises are outward signs of a more serious internal injury or medical condition. Contact your doctor if your child develops bruises that aren't the result of an obvious bump or mishap; spontaneous bruising can indicate a nutritional deficiency or a serious illness such as anemia or leukemia.

In addition, you should contact a doctor if the bruise appears on the head or eye, if a fever develops, if your child becomes drowsy and one pupil is larger than the other, or if your child has trouble walking or talking or reports a vision problem.

Burns

Children don't understand your frantic warnings—''Stop, that's hot!''—until they experience their first burn. While most parents think of burns as caused by heat, they can also be caused by corrosive chemicals or electricity.

After a child has been burned, your first step should be to remove the cause, by removing the heat, washing away the chemicals, or eliminating the source of electricity. You'll need to assess the severity of the burn to determine treatment. Burns can be divided into three levels of intensity:

- First-degree burns, which cause the skin to turn red and feel tender;
- Second-degree burns, which cause the skin to blister and peel; and
- Third-degree burns, which devour all layers of the skin and destroy the nerve endings, leaving charred and burned tissue behind.

While painful and unpleasant, first-degree burns rarely pose any medical risk and usually can be treated at home. Second-degree burns should be seen by a doctor to minimize the risk of infection, especially if the burns are extensive, but these burns rarely cause scarring or lead to any significant medical problems. Third-degree burns should be considered medical emergencies and treated by a medical professional immediately.

Traditional Treatments

Cool it. Immediately apply cold water. The faster you can cool the area, the less skin damage will result from the burn. Submerge the burned area in cold water for 5–10 minutes, then check to see that the area is not being numbed from the cold. Reapply the cold as necessary. Cold water is more effective than ice, in addition to being gentler on the skin.

Forget the butter. The old wives' tale of applying butter to a burn does nothing to treat the burn—and may make the problem worse. The butter does not help cool the area and can trap the heat under the skin, where it causes more extensive tissue damage. Leave the butter in the fridge and turn the cold water on instead.

Treat the pain. Burns can be excruciatingly painful. Give your child acetaminophen to ease the pain and reduce the swelling. Of course, never give a child under age 18 aspirin (including ''baby aspirin''), due to the risk of developing Reye's syndrome, a potentially fatal disorder.

If it ain't broke . . . If blisters develop, leave them alone. The blister protects the damaged skin underneath and reduces the risk of infection. If the blisters break naturally, wash the area thoroughly and leave the skin flap in place. Cover the area with a sterile gauze pad and keep it scrupulously clean.

Natural Remedies

All of the natural remedies listed below can be used to supplement conventional medical treatment.

Diet and Nutrition

Use one or more of the remedies listed below. Dosage varies according to age; see the chart on pages 14–15 to determine to correct dose for your child. Some vitamins can be used topically, as noted. For good food sources of particular nutrients, see pages 9–13.

• A cool compress of whole milk soothes the burns and promotes healing. Soak a clean cloth in chilled whole milk and apply it to the burn site for 15 or 20 minutes, then rinse thoroughly.

- Vitamins A and E help speed the healing process. Give your child 1 dose of vitamins A and E 2 times a day for 3 or 4 days. In addition, apply vitamin E oil directly to the burn 3 or 4 times a day to help prevent scarring.
- Vitamin C promotes healing of burns and other wounds. Give your child 1 dose of vitamin C 3 times a day for 3 or 4 days.

Herbal

Use one or more of the topical remedies listed below. Allow the skin to dry between applications, if you want to use more than one treatment at the same time.

- Aloe can relieve the stinging pain of a burn and speed the healing process by as much as 40 percent. Just snap off a leaf of this cactus-like plant and apply the gel directly to the burn site. Reapply as many times as necessary throughout the day, for as long as needed. Commercially prepared aloe treatments are also available.
- Calendula ointment can help prevent infection at the burn site. Apply the ointment directly to the burn site twice a day for 2 or 3 days.
- Lavender helps ease the pain of minor burns. Dilute 5–6 drops of lavender oil in a teaspoon of lotion and gently rub the solution into the burn. Repeat 2 or 3 times a day for as long as necessary.
- Tea tree oil cools the burn and soothes the pain. Apply it directly to the burn 2 or 3 times daily for as long as necessary.

Homeopathy

Use one homeopathic treatment at a time, based on your child's specific symptoms. For dosage information, see the chart on pages 31–37. Discontinue use if the symptoms disappear.

- *Arnica (Arnica montana)* 30c: Use for all burns. Give 1 dose every 15 minutes as soon as the burn or scald has been cooled, for up to 3 doses.

- *Hepar sulph. (Hepar sulphuris calcareum)* 6c: Use if a burn becomes infected. Give 1 dose every 4 hours, up to 10 doses.
- *Kali bichrom. (Kali bichromicum)* 6c: Use on second-degree burns. Give 1 dose every 4 hours, for up to 10 doses.
- *Urtica (Urtica wrens)* 6c: Use if the burn continues to sting. Give 1 dose every 15 minutes, for up to 6 doses.

An Ounce of Prevention

Sit down with your family and review the basics of fire safety. Install smoke alarms throughout your home; do not allow your children to play with matches; stage a ''fire drill'' to teach your children how to respond in case of fire; store flammable substances in appropriate places. In addition, prevent burns by turning the handles on your pots and pans toward the back of the stove (away from little hands), and set the thermostat on the hot water heater to no more than 120 degrees F. (At 140 degrees F, water can cause a third-degree burn in as little as five seconds; at 120 degrees F, it would take 3 minutes to cause a comparable burn.)

When to Call for Help

All serious burns demand a doctor's attention. Take your child to the doctor if a burn blisters or turns the skin white, if a burn covers more than 10 percent of your child's body, if a burn remains painful after 48 hours, or if a burn involves the mouth, face, hands, or genitals. In addition, call your doctor if a burn appears swollen, oozes pus, or shows other signs of infection.

Canker Sores

If you've ever had a canker sore, you know just what your canker sore-afflicted little one is going through when he cringes at the thought of drinking his orange juice or pushes his plate away when confronted with a fresh fruit salad.

Canker sores (*aphthous ulcers*) are little red sores with white or yellow centers that usually show up on the mouth or gums. They form when mouth acids and digestive enzymes eat away the soft tissue of the mouth. For some reason, certain unfortunate people are far more prone than others to experience outbreaks, which usually last 4 or 5 days. These oral ulcers can be caused or aggravated by certain foods (mentioned later), stress, or minor mouth injuries and skin irritation. Unlike cold sores (see page 111), canker sores cannot be spread from person to person.

Traditional Treatments

- *Wash your kid's mouth out.* Ask your child to rinse his mouth out with warm water frequently throughout the day to keep the area clean. Crush a Tums or Rolaids tablet and apply the powder to the sore to neutralize the acid that causes the discomfort. Another option: Dilute 1 tablespoon of hydrogen peroxide in ½ cup of water and have your child swish the solution around in his mouth to disinfect the sore and speed healing. NOTE: Only use hydrogen peroxide with a child old enough not to swallow the solution.
- *What pain?* Ease the pain with a Popsicle, an ice cube, or an anesthetic lozenge. These remedies may not last long, but they can provide fast, temporary relief.
- *Watch what goes in the mouth.* Canker sores can be made worse by nuts, coconut, candy bars, and chocolate. These

treats may be tempting, but explain that they can make existing sores feel worse, and in some children they also may cause sores to form. When your child has a sore, avoid giving him fruit juices, citrus fruits, and acidic foods, which can really hurt when they make contact with the open wound.

Natural Remedies

All of the natural remedies listed below can be used to supplement conventional medical treatment.

Diet and Nutrition

Use one or more of the remedies listed below. Dosage varies according to age; see the chart on pages 14–15 to determine to correct dose for your child. Some vitamins can be used topically, as noted. For good food sources of particular nutrients, see pages 9–13.

- Avoid hot, spicy, and acidic foods, which can irritate the lining of the mouth. Encourage your child to pass on the Mexican food and three-alarm chili, as well as tomatoes and citrus fruits, which can be acidic.
- Have your child take a one-a-day vitamin. Canker sores have been linked to deficiencies of certain nutrients, including iron and vitamin B_{12}.
- Apply several drops of vitamin E oil directly on the canker sore. Repeat several times a day.
- Zinc will boost the immune system and ease the pain of canker sores. Give your child a zinc lozenge and have him hold it against the sore 2 or 3 times a day.

Herbal

Use one or more of the remedies listed below. Dosage varies according to age; see the chart on page 25 to determine the correct dose for your child.

- Black tea contains tannin, an astringent that has pain-relieving ability. Hold a wet, black tea bag against the sore for 10 minutes, 2 or 3 times a day.
- Make a paste using a teaspoon of goldenseal powder and a few drops of water and apply it directly to the ulcer. Do this daily until the sore disappears.
- Licorice root has antiviral and antibacterial properties, and it can ease the irritation of a canker sore. Make licorice root tea and have your child swish the warm liquid around in his mouth once or twice a day.

Acupressure

For a diagram showing the specific pressure points, see pages 40–41.

- Bigger Rushing (Liver 3): This point is located on top of the foot in the valley between the big toe and the second toe.

An Ounce of Prevention

Since no one knows exactly what causes canker sores, it's impossible to offer surefire ways of preventing them. However, you can reduce the number of sores your child must live with by encouraging your child to avoid sharp, hard-bristled toothbrushes, rotary toothbrushes, and other objects that can injure or irritate the lining of the mouth. In addition, a daily helping of yogurt can help keep the lining of the mouth healthy and ward off canker sores and other mouth infections.

When to Call for Help

Canker sores should heal within two weeks. If your child has a long-lasting sore or a recurrent sore, contact your doctor or dentist. Your child may need an antibiotic, or the doctor may need to cauterize the sore. In addition, a sharp edge to a tooth or another dental problem could aggravate a canker sore and not give it a chance to heal.

Sometimes canker sores come in clusters and spread along the back of the throat. The bad news: This condition, known as herpangina, is extremely painful. The good news: Once your child has herpangina, he won't get it a second time. The virus can be treated with the same methods as other canker sores, but you might want to contact your doctor if the sores don't start to disappear within 4 or 5 days.

Chicken Pox

Your child complains of a fever and sluggishness. Probably a cold, you think. Then a spot shows up on his back, probably a bug bite, you think. Next time you look, your little one is covered with tiny red spots and the reality is undeniable: Your child has the chicken pox.

The disease will usually run its course in about a week or so, and in the process your child will have to deal with blisters, itching, and scabbing. In general, the older the person, the more uncomfortable the symptoms, though outbreaks can be mild or severe at any age.

Chicken pox is caused by a virus (*Varicella zoster*) that stays in the system and can manifest itself later as shingles in both adults and children. The virus is very contagious, and it usually shows up 1–3 weeks after your child has been exposed to the virus. After a day or so of low fever, your child's temperature may rise and he may begin to show his spots; additional marks usually appear for the next 3 or 4 days. The spots start out as red marks, usually appearing on the trunk, armpits, scalp, and inside the mouth. The spots then form clear blisters, which pop, leaving behind a scab. In the final stage of the illness, the fever drops off and the scabs begin to heal.

Your child can spread the disease from a day before the spots appear to the time the last of the blisters scabs over. Shallow scars or pockmarks may be left when the scabs fall off, but these spots usually fill in over time, unless your child has scratched the area and caused skin damage.

Traditional Treatments

- *Cool the fever.* If your child is burning up with fever and generally achy and uncomfortable, look in the medicine cabinet for some acetaminophen. Check the package for directions for the correct dosage. Don't bother about fighting the fever if your child can tolerate it, since it may help shorten the duration of the disease. WARNING: Never give aspirin (or "baby aspirin") to a child under age 18 with chicken pox because it can cause Reye's syndrome, a potentially fatal disease.

- *Dress for success.* Dress your child in light cotton clothes, especially in the first 2–3 days of the disease. Heat will irritate the pox and cause more itching.

- *Time for a cold shower.* Or a least a cool bath filled with an anti-itch agent, such as an oatmeal treatment. Aveeno oatmeal is available in most pharmacies (follow package directions for proper use). Consider adding ½ cup of baking soda to the bath water if oatmeal isn't available. The baths not only help with itching, but they also keep the skin clean, which can minimize the risk of infection.

- *Look, don't touch.* Try to discourage your child from scratching the pox, but understand that the urge will be intense. Clip your child's nails as short as possible to decrease risk of infection and scarring. Have your child scrub his fingernails frequently with soap and water to prevent a secondary infection.

- *A little dab will do ya.* If some of the sores look red or pus-filled, dab a little over-the-counter antibiotic ointment on the area.

- *When willpower isn't enough.* If your child has trouble resisting the urge to scratch, help him out by giving him an over-the-counter antihistamine. (Follow package directions for appropriate dosage.) You might also try calamine lotion with phenol, a topical anesthetic. At night, consider having him wear mittens to avoid scratching in his sleep.

- *Don't make a bad situation worse.* Don't use any over-the-counter hydrocortisone creams, even though they claim to fight the itch. The steroids can inhibit the immune system from dealing with the virus.
- *Don't let the sun shine.* Avoid the rays when your child has chicken pox; the skin can become sunburned much faster when battling the virus than at other times. If your child can't stay indoors, apply a sunscreen with a sun protection factor (SPF) of 15 or higher, even on the pox themselves. This increased sun sensitivity doesn't disappear with the pockmarks; your child's skin will remain tender for about a year.

Natural Remedies

All of the natural remedies listed below can be used to supplement conventional medical treatment.

Diet and Nutrition
Use one or more of the remedies listed below. Dosage varies according to age; see the chart on pages 14–15 to determine the correct dose for your child. Some vitamins can be used topically, as noted. For good food sources of particular nutrients, see pages 9–13.

- Be sure your child drinks plenty of fluids. Fever can cause dehydration.
- Vitamin A stimulates the immune system and assists with tissue healing. Give your child 1 dose every day for 10 days.
- Rub vitamin E oil or cream directly on the pox, provided the skin is not broken.

Herbal
Use one or more of the remedies listed below. Dosage varies according to age; see the chart on page 25 to determine the correct dose for your child.

- Apply aloe vera gel directly to the affected skin to ease the itching.

- Mix 4 teaspoons of bicarbonate of soda with ½ gallon of warm water and use as a compress to help the pox dry and heal.
- Give your child chamomile tea to help him relax and sleep.
- Give your child oatmeal baths using Aveeno powder (available at pharmacies) to minimize itching.

Homeopathy

Use one homeopathic treatment at a time, based on your child's specific symptoms. For dosage information, see the chart on pages 31–37. Discontinue use if the symptoms disappear.

- *Belladonna (Atropa belladonna)* 30c: Use if your child has a low fever and general achiness. Give 1 dose every 2 hours for up to 8 doses when the red spots first appear.
- *Mercurius (Mercurius solubilis hahnemanni)* 6c: Use if your child's temperature is down and the spots are beginning to heal but some are still infected. Give 1 dose every 2 hours for up to 8 doses.
- *Pulsatilla (Pulsatilla nigricans)* 6c: Use if your child has a rash and fever. Give 1 dose every 2 hours for up to 8 doses.
- *Rhus tox. (Rhus toxicodendron)* 30c: Use if your child has been exposed to another child with chicken pox. Give 1 dose a day for 10 days as a preventive measure.
- *Sulphur* 30x or 9c: Use if your child's spots are very red and itchy. Give 1 dose 3 times a day for up to 3 days.

Acupressure

Use one or more of the acupressure points listed below. For a diagram showing the specific pressure points, see pages 40–41.

- Crooked Pond (Large Intestine 11): Apply steady pressure on the point located at the top, outer edge of the elbow crease.
- Joining the Valley (Large Intestine 4): This point is located in the webbing between your thumb and index finger. On the outside of the hand, find the highest spot of the muscle where the thumb and index fingers are brought closest together.

An Ounce of Prevention

Until recently, parents couldn't do much to prevent their children from coming down with chicken pox. However, the U.S. Food and Drug Administration recently approved a chicken pox vaccine. Talk to your doctor about it.

When to Call for Help

Most cases of chicken pox come and go without complication, but the virus has been linked to encephalitis and Reye's syndrome, both of which are life-threatening brain inflammations. (Complications are more common in adults.) Call your child's pediatrician if the fever persists after the pox have scabbed over, if your child experiences neck pain, or if your child has severe headache, vomiting, disorientation, or convulsions.

Other less serious complications are also possible. Call the doctor if your child has a number of swollen, painful sores that look infected, if your child develops an earache, sore throat, or chronic cough. Vaginal or rectal sores may also require a doctor's attention.

Colds

There's no getting around it: Your kid is going to get sick—and often—as he faces the lifetime challenge of building a strong immune system. More than two hundred different viruses cause colds, and your child has to build immunity to them one by one. That explains why kids catch 6–10 colds a year. (By adulthood your child will have been exposed to many of the cold viruses out there, which is why most adults catch only 2–4 colds a year.)

Technically speaking, a cold is a viral infection of the upper respiratory tract, which includes the nose, throat, sinuses, and bronchial tubes. When confronted with the viral invaders, the nose and throat release chemicals to stoke up the immune system. The affected cells produce prostaglandins, which stimulate inflammation and lure the infection-fighting white blood cells. The body temperature rises to boost the immune response and more nasal mucus is produced to trap and wash away viral particles.

Inside your child's nasal passages, a battle is waged between the evil virus and the virtuous, infection-fighting white blood cells: It's not the virus itself, but the body's defenses that make your child feel lousy. In fact, the virus has been in the body for about 24 hours before your child even begins to feel he's coming down with a cold.

Since viruses cause colds—and antibiotics don't work against viruses—when your child comes down with a cold the best you can do is to treat the symptoms. Colds are self-limiting: They last about a week, no matter what you do. (Remember the adage, "Treat a cold and it'll last a week; leave it alone and it will last seven days.") All you can really do when your child has a cold is provide comfort, deal with his symptoms one by one, and wait patiently for the virus to be overpowered by the immune system.

Traditional Treatments

Replenish the fluids. Drinking fluids helps to prevent dehydration and to thin nasal mucus, reducing the risk of ear infection and sinus problems. Warm soup and beverages help relieve congestion, and they soothe a sore throat. And, yes, chicken soup really does help. A study conducted at Mt. Sinai Hospital in Miami Beach found that chicken soup was more effective than hot water or cold water at clearing away nasal mucus.

Rest, nap, and lounge. One of the best ways to boost the immune system and cut short the down time with a cold is to get plenty of rest. During periods of rest (and your child doesn't need to be sleeping to be resting), the body releases compounds that enhance the immune system.

Monitor the fever. You'll want to keep an eye on your child's fever to make sure it doesn't get too high, but a low fever can actually help your child get better faster because it mobilizes the immune system and helps fight infection. How high is too high? Take steps to lower a child's fever at 100 degrees. (Contact a doctor if your child is below age 3 and has a fever of 102 degrees or higher, or above age 3 and has a fever of 104 degrees or higher.) To bring down the fever, give your child acetaminophen, following the package directions for the appropriate dosage. And never give your child under age 18 aspirin (or "baby aspirin") due to the risk of Reye's syndrome, a potentially fatal brain and liver disorder.

Treat the symptoms. When your child has a cold, your challenge will be to deal with each of your child's complaints. For advice on coughing, see page 125; for fever, see page 160; for runny nose, see page 246; for sore throat, see page 250; and for stuffy nose, see page 263. If you want to try an over-the-counter cold remedy for children, avoid using multi-action products because they tend to overmedicate by giving your child drugs to control symptoms he may not have. (Most cold symptoms occur serially, not simultaneously.) Instead, deal with the symptoms one by one.

Natural Remedies

All of the natural remedies listed below can be used to supplement conventional medical treatment.

Diet and Nutrition

Use one or more of the remedies listed below. Dosage varies according to age; see the chart on pages 14–15 to determine to correct dose for your child. For good food sources of particular nutrients, see pages 9–13.

- Vitamin A helps fight infection and boost the immune system. Give your child 1 dose of vitamin A twice a day for 5 days.
- Vitamin C helps reduce inflammation and boost the immune system. Give your child 1 dose of vitamin C 3–

4 times a day for 5 days, beginning at the first hint of cold
symptoms.
- Zinc boosts the immune system and helps fight off certain
common cold viruses. If your child is old enough to suck
on a lozenge without choking, give your child up to 3 zinc
lozenges a day for 3 or 4 days.

Herbal
Use one or more of the remedies listed below. Dosage varies
according to age; see the chart on page 25 to determine the
correct dose for your child.

- Chamomile tea will help your child rest and relax. Give your
child 1 dose twice daily, as needed.
- Echinacea boosts the immune system and helps fight viral
infection. Give your child 1 dose of echinacea once a day,
or as directed on the package label.
- Garlic helps fight infection and speed healing. Give your
child 2 or 3 doses of odorless garlic a day, or follow package
directions.
- Licorice tea soothes a sore throat and helps relieve coughs.
Give your child 3 doses a day for 3 or 4 days.

Homeopathy
Use one homeopathic treatment at a time, based on your
child's specific symptoms. For dosage information, see the
chart on pages 31–37. Discontinue use if the symptoms disappear.

- *Aconite (Aconitum napellus)* 30c: Use if your child develops
sneezing, burning throat, and other cold symptoms suddenly,
especially after exposure to cold temperatures. Give 1 dose
every 2 hours for up to 4 doses.
- *Allium (Allium cepa)* 12x or 6c: Use if your child has a very
runny nose and nasal inflammation. Give 1 dose 3 times
daily for 3 days.
- *Euphrasia (Euphrasia officinalis)* 12x: Use if your child has
irritated and burning eyes, especially at night. Give 1 dose
3 times daily for 3 days.
- *Gelsemium (Gelsemium sempervirens)* 30x or 9c: Use if

your child feels sluggish and tired and has heavy eyes. Give 1 dose 3 times daily for 3 days.

Acupressure

Use one or more of the acupressure points listed below. For a diagram showing the specific pressure points, see pages 40–41.

- Drilling Bamboo (Bladder 2): This point is located in the indentations of the eye sockets, on either side of where the bridge of the nose meets the ridge of the eyebrows.
- Facial ·Beauty (Stomach 3): To find this point, place your fingers at the bottom of the cheekbones, directly below the pupil.
- Heavenly Rejuvenation (Triple Warmer 15): Apply steady pressure on the point on the shoulders, midway between the base of the neck and the outside of the shoulders, ½ inch below the top of the shoulders.
- Third Eye Point (Governing Vessel 24.5): This point is located directly between the eyebrows, in the indentation where the bridge of the nose meets the center of the forehead.

An Ounce of Prevention

You can't prevent your child from catching every cold, but you may be able to decrease the odds of catching every one that's going around by practicing good hand-washing habits. The stronger your child's immune system, the more likely he can shake off a cold, so try to feed your child a balanced diet and keep him well rested.

If your child is breast-feeding, keep it up. Breast-feeding provides extra protection against cold viruses because some of the mother's immunities pass on to the baby through the breast milk. Mom should continue breast-feeding if she has a cold, though she should make a point to drink extra fluids to remain fully hydrated.

When to Call for Help

Most colds don't require a visit to the doctor. After all, there's nothing your doctor can do to make the cold disappear any faster than it will on its own. However, you should call the pediatrician if your child develops an earache, shortness of breath, or a fever that lingers for several days (which could indicate a bacterial infection rather than a cold).

In addition, if the sinus pain and congestion don't clear up within ten days, call the doctor. The blocked nasal passages may have created a sinus infection, which should be treated with prescription antibiotics. Because of their small nasal passages, sinus infections are common in young children. In fact, fully 90 percent of children under age 6 who have congestion for more than 10 days have developed a sinus infection.

Cold Sores

Cold sores show up at the most inopportune times: before the prom, on exam day, or during the holidays. Sometimes cold sores (also called fever blisters) show up once and never return, other times they repeatedly return, subjecting some unfortunate children to unkind remarks from classmates.

Cold sores are caused by the herpes simplex virus, a close relative of the virus that causes genital herpes. There's not much you can do to prevent your child from encountering the highly contagious virus. In fact, most people are exposed to it by their fifth birthday, even if they don't show signs of infection. It can be passed on by a loving kiss from Grandma, by a handshake with a stranger, or by sharing blocks with another kid in kindergarten.

The virus can cause fatigue and fever for a week or two, then it may lay dormant in a nerve, never to be heard from again. For about 1 in 10 children, however, the virus will cause blisters to form on the lips, chin, gums, or fingers. These blisters break open, ooze, then form a yellowish sore. In a week or so, the sore dries up and fades away. For some kids, the nightmare is over after a single outbreak, but other kids will suffer from repeated outbreaks throughout their lives.

Traditional Treatments

- *Heed the herpes warning.* Before a cold sore appears, most people experience a tingly feeling in the lips and face where the breakout will occur. Encourage your child to take this warning seriously and apply over-the-counter cold sore drops to the site. These drops contain tannic acid, which can either minimize or wipe out the sore before it has a chance to show its ugly face. The earlier you tend to the sore, the more effective the treatment will be; you usually have 4–8 hours to zap it for treatment to be of any use.
- *Keep it moist.* To avoid dry, cracked skin, moisturize the sore and the area around it by using petroleum jelly or another ointment that will trap the moisture under the skin. Reapply as often as needed.
- *Keep your hands to yourself.* Touching the sore can cause a bacterial infection, which can spread the disease to other parts of the body or to unsuspecting friends and family members. Encourage your child to leave the sore alone, and give him something to keep busy. If your child touches the sore, have him thoroughly wash his hands with soap and water.
- *Time for a new toothbrush.* Trash your child's toothbrush at the first sign of an outbreak. The virus can live in a toothbrush for days, reinfecting your child when the initial sore shows signs of healing. Once the sore disappears, replace the toothbrush a second time.

Natural Remedies

All of the natural remedies listed below can be used to supplement conventional medical treatment.

Diet and Nutrition
Use one or more of the remedies listed below. Dosage varies according to age; see the chart on pages 14–15 to determine to correct dose for your child. For good food sources of particular nutrients, see pages 9–13.

- Folic acid heals the mucous membranes. Give your child 1 dose a day until the sore disappears.
- Lactobacillus acidophilus helps cure existing cold sores and prevent new ones from breaking out. Take 1 dose of live bacteria a day, following package instructions.
- Vitamin C with bioflavonoids can help cure cold sores. Give your child 1 dose daily.

Herbal
Use one or more of the remedies listed below. Dosage varies according to age; see the chart on page 25 to determine the correct dose for your child.

- Garlic helps fight viruses, including the virus that causes cold sores. Give your child 1 dose of odorless garlic twice a day until the sore disappears.
- Sprinkle powdered marjoram on the sores several times a day to inhibit the growth of the virus.
- Moisten a tea bag with warm water and hold it against the tingly area before an outbreak occurs. Tea contains tannic acid, which has antiviral properties that can minimize the size of the sore or keep it from appearing at all. Hold the tea bag in place for 5 minutes every hour, for up to 12 hours.

Homeopathy
Use one homeopathic treatment at a time, based on your child's specific symptoms. For dosage information, see the chart on pages 31–37. Discontinue use if the symptoms disappear.

- *Capsicum (Capsicum annuum)* 6c: Use if your child has cracks at the corners of his mouth and an itchy rash on his chin. Give 1 dose 4 times daily for up to 5 days.
- *Rhus tox. (Rhus toxicodendron)* 6c: Use if your child's

mouth and chin are infected. Give 1 dose 4 times daily for up to 5 days.

An Ounce of Prevention

Once your child harbors the herpes cold sore virus, there is a chance that the virus will strike again. Generally, cold sores surface when your child is sick, stressed, or unrested. Sunburn and wind can also exacerbate breakouts, so be sure your child wears sunscreen and lip balm with a sun protection factor (SPF) of 15 or higher, and blocks the winter cold with a warm scarf, high-necked coat, and ski mask.

When to Call for Help

Though they are annoying and unattractive, most cold sores aren't serious enough to require a visit to the doctor. There are, however, a few exceptions. Notify your doctor if the cold sore lingers for more than two weeks, if there are a number of sores in and around the mouth, or if your child is younger than 1 year old.

Colic

All babies fuss and cry, sometimes sobbing for an hour or more before quieting down and falling asleep. But that's not colic. No, as parents of babes with colic can tell you, if your little one has colic, you'll know it. Colic is characterized by inconsolable, rhythmic wailing and anguished crying that drags on for 3–4 hours at a time—or longer. The exasperating part for parents is that no matter what they do, it's generally not good enough to silence the cry.

Colic usually shows up when a baby is 2–6 weeks old and fades within about 3 months, though it can linger for up to 4 or 5 months. Colic occurs in healthy babies and has no long-term negative effects. With most babies, the fussy periods settle into a somewhat predictable pattern, such as crying that starts around 7 P.M. and lasts for several hours.

Though as many as 20 percent of babies develop colic, doctors don't know exactly what causes it. Some argue that an immature digestive system contributes to the problem, especially since many colicky babies clench their fists and draw their legs up tight to the tummy as though they're in great abdominal pain. Sometimes the crying bouts come before or after bowel movements. Other experts blame colic on food allergies and nervous system development. The upshot is that no one knows exactly what causes the problem, or exactly how to deal with it. That leaves parents with the trial-and-error course of treatment—and the knowledge that sooner or later this too shall pass.

Traditional Treatments

If at first you don't succeed . . . When it comes to managing colic, you'll have to experiment with a number of techniques, in hopes of stumbling into one that works for your child. Of course, start with the basics: Make sure your child is clean, fed, comfortable, and comforted. If all your child's fundamental needs have been met and he's still wailing, let the experimenting begin. Try an approach for just 5 or 10 minutes; if it doesn't work, give up and switch to something else.

Let's dance. Some children respond to music and motion. Try putting on some music and waltzing around the room. If your kid doesn't like classical, try rock or jazz or the blues. (Even if your kid keeps crying, the music may help you work out some of your own frustration.)

White noise may be the right noise. Loud, humming noises and gentle vibration can soothe the frazzled spirit of a colicky little one. Try putting your baby in a front-pack and vacuuming the carpets, or strapping him in the car seat and going for a joy ride.

Try a warm snuggle. Warmth can help soothe muscle cramps and calm a colicky infant. Hold your child against your chest with a warm water bottle between you and your baby. The gentle warmth can be relaxing to some infants, but be careful not to let the baby get overheated, since it can cause prickly heat and make your child uncomfortable.

Work out those bubbles. Moving your baby's legs can help stimulate the digestive system and work out painful gas bubbles. Place your baby on his back on the bed and gently move his legs around in a bicycle-pedaling motion.

Sometimes less is more. Too much stimulation can cause some infants to switch into overload, screaming and crying just to shut of the rest of the world. If your baby goes nuts when you try to comfort him, he may need to be left alone. Rocking or singing to an overstimulated child will only make matters worse. Put your baby in the crib and let him cry for 10 or 15 minutes. He may calm down on his own, but if he doesn't, try something else.

Burp, excuse me. Be sure to burp or "bubble" your baby often during feeding to minimize the risk of air bubbles getting trapped in your child's digestive system, causing gas pain. The less air that goes in, the less trouble with the air coming out. Keep your child in an upright position during feeding, and if you use a bottle, make sure the nipple holes are the appropriate size (it should drip slowly when held upside down).

Escape. Parents of colicky children experience tremendous stress and frustration, on top of the usual sleep deprivation and challenges of adjusting to a new baby. Get help with child care; you need a break and reassurance from someone who can remind you that colic is a temporary medical condition, not a sign that you are an inadequate parent. Talk to other parents; join a colic support group; hire an experienced baby-sitter and go shopping or read at the public library for the afternoon.

Natural Remedies

All of the natural remedies listed below can be used to supplement conventional medical treatment.

Diet and Nutrition
Use one or more of the remedies listed below.

- Some breast-fed babies are sensitive to foods that their mothers eat. Common culprits include dairy products, beans, broccoli, chocolate, caffeine, cucumbers, citrus fruits, onions, and spicy foods. Try eliminating these foods from the diet one by one to see if they are causing the problem.
- Breast-feeding mothers should take Lactobacillus acidophilus to boost the levels of beneficial bacteria in the intestinal system. A breast-feeding mother can take ½ teaspoon twice a day; bottle-fed babies can have ½ teaspoon mixed in with the formula twice a day.

Herbal
Use one or more of the remedies listed below.

- Chamomile tea promotes relaxation. To soothe a colicky infant, a breast-feeding mother should drink one cup twice a day. Bottle-fed infants can have 1 teaspoon of tea mixed with formula twice a day, for 2 or 3 days.
- Fennel may help ease colic pain. A breast-feeding mother can drink one cup of fennel tea twice a day. *Fennel tea should not be given directly to infants.*
- Peppermint tea helps with digestion and relieves gas pain. Whether breast-feeding or bottle-feeding, give your child 1 teaspoon of peppermint tea 3 times a day for as long as necessary.

Homeopathy
Use one homeopathic treatment at a time, based on your child's specific symptoms. For dosage information, see the chart on pages 31–37. Discontinue use if the symptoms disappear.

- *Carbo veg. (Carbo vegetabilis)* 12x or 9c: Use if your child feels better when held, and cries when being fed. Give 1 dose every 5 minutes for up to 10 doses.

- *Chamomilla (Chamomilla vulgaris)* 6c: Use if your baby is impossible to please, but seems to improve when carried around. Give 1 dose every 5 minutes for up to 10 doses.
- *Colocynth (Citrullus colocynthis)* 12x or 6c: Use if the crying is relieved by firm pressure on stomach. Give 1 dose every 5 minutes for up to 10 doses.

Acupressure
Use one or more of the acupressure points listed below. For a diagram showing the specific pressure points, see pages 40–41.

- Abdominal Sorrow (Spleen 16): This point is located below the edge of the rib cage ½ inch in from the nipple line.
- Sea of Energy (Conception Vessel 6): To find this point, place your fingers 2 child's finger widths directly below belly button.
- Three Mile Point (Stomach 36): Apply steady pressure on the point 4 child's finger widths below the kneecap toward the outside of the shinbone.

An Ounce of Prevention

Colic can't be prevented, though you may be able to reduce some gastrointestinal discomfort by burping your baby often and trying to keep feeding time as calm and quiet as possible.

When to Call for Help

With a newborn, you will be visiting the doctor every few weeks for checkups and immunizations, so you will have plenty of opportunities to discuss the problem with a physician. Don't hesitate to ask for help and seek reassurance from your doctor.

Concussion and Head Injury

All head injuries should be taken seriously, even though few will actually result in serious problems. With head injuries that don't involve obvious damage to the skull, the primary concern is internal bleeding, which can result in pressure on the brain and damage to the delicate tissues. If your child suffers a fall, a blow to the head, or a sudden jarring or shaking, call your doctor and observe your child's behavior carefully. Don't be surprised if heavy bleeding accompanies a head injury because the head is replete with blood vessels.

Traditional Treatments

If your child suffers a head injury, after alerting your doctor, wrap ice in a clean cloth and apply it to the bruised area to minimize swelling.

Depending on the severity of the injury, your doctor may recommend that you observe your child and call again if symptoms appear, usually within the first 1–3 days. (Symptoms of a concussion are listed below.) Check on your child every 2 hours during the first day, every 4 hours during the second day, and every 8 hours during the third day. Keep in mind that the more severe the injury, the longer it can take for symptoms to appear.

Natural Remedies

All of the natural remedies listed below can be used to supplement conventional medical treatment.

Homeopathy

Use one homeopathic treatment at a time, based on your child's specific symptoms. For dosage information, see the chart on pages 31–37. Discontinue use if the symptoms disappear.

- *Aconite (Aconitum napellus)* 200x: To alleviate some of the initial shock, administer 1 dose immediately after the accident.
- *Arnica (Arnica montana)* 30x, 200x, 15c or 30c: 1 dose given immediately after the injury occurs helps to decrease bruising and aching. Give 1 dose 3 times a day for 2 days following the accident.

An Ounce of Prevention

Some accidents cannot be prevented, but others can. Teach your child about bicycle safety and demand that he wear a crash-tested helmet approved by either the American National Standards Institute (ANSI) or the Snell Memorial Foundation. The vast majority of bicycle-related deaths and serious injuries are due to head injury, and 85 percent of bicycle-related head injuries can be prevented by wearing helmets. Also make sure your child wears a helmet when playing hockey and football, skateboarding, and participating in other potentially risky behaviors.

In addition, treat your child gently. Never shake him, especially in anger. Do not toss him in the air and catch him. Both practices can cause brain stem injury.

When to Call for Help

Head injuries are one of the most common causes of death in children. Call your physician after any head injury, or visit the hospital emergency room. It can be very difficult to assess the severity of a head injury, so always seek professional medical help.

Symptoms of concussion and the need for emergency care

include shallow breathing, nausea, unusually wide or uneven pupils, drowsiness, loss of consciousness (even for several seconds), brief loss of memory, confusion, and cold, clammy skin.

Constipation

All babies grunt, grimace, and turn red-faced when having a bowel movement. All this hard work doesn't necessarily mean your child is constipated. When children grow up and no longer make such an obvious spectacle of their bathroom habits, they might wait as much as a week between bowel movements. This infrequency concerns some parents, but it doesn't necessarily mean your child is constipated.

Constipation involves difficult and painful bowel movements, regardless of what "normal" frequency is for your child. If your child is constipated, he probably strains to pass dry, hard stools, and may complain of gas pains or bloating. In severe cases, the bowel may become impacted and stop moving through the digestive tract.

Constipation usually stems from dietary problems, such as dehydration or a lack of fiber in the diet, though toddlers sometimes develop constipation for emotional reasons, especially during the toilet-training process. (One thing you can't make your child do is move his bowels, and your child knows this is one area where you're not in control.) Still, with a few simple changes in diet and lifestyle, your child's constipation should clear right up.

Traditional Treatments

Drink up. When it comes to constipation, the simplest solution is to encourage your child to drink more fluids. Offer water and fruit juice, which can loosen the bowels. (Even infants can drink apple juice once it has been introduced into the diet.) The extra water will be of particular importance when you supplement your child's diet with high-fiber foods, which tend to absorb water to form soft stools.

Add fiber. High-fiber foods help keep the digestive system moving along smoothly. Supplement your child's diet with high-fiber foods, such as fruits, vegetables, whole wheat breads, and bran. Bake a batch of bran muffins with raisins for breakfast and offer carrots and raw vegetables (perhaps with peanut butter) as a crunchy between-meal snack.

Know what to eat. Some foods tend to be binding and contribute to hard stools. If your child is constipated, cut back on the bananas, applesauce, and white rice, which can make stools harder and drier.

Exercise. Regular exercise promotes regular bowel movements. Encourage your child to go for a walk after dinner or a bike ride in the afternoon. With an infant, you can lie the baby on his back on the bed and move his legs through the bicycle motion to exercise the limbs and stimulate the bowels.

Make time for potty. Some kids would rather keep on playing a game or watching television than stopping the action long enough to use the toilet. The result can be constipation or an impacted bowel. If your child has trouble listening to his body's needs, at regular intervals stop the play and insist that your child sit on the toilet for 5–10 minutes, whether he says he needs to go or not.

Talk to your pharmacist. A number of over-the-counter products help relieve constipation in babies and children, but they should be used only occasionally to avoid creating dependence. First try diet and exercise. If that doesn't work, consider glycerin suppositories for infants and young children, or an over-the-counter laxative for older children. Follow the package directions for dosage information.

''You're in charge.'' Toddlers strive to exercise control over their lives, and toilet training and bowel movements are one of the favorite arenas for kids to challenge parental authority. To minimize the battle of wills, avoid starting on toilet training before your child shows signs of readiness, often closer to age three than age two. Try to shift the battleground from the bathroom (where your child will try to express control by

withholding bowel movements) to the bedroom (where your child will try to express control by choosing which clothes to wear or how to arrange the stuffed animals on the bed). Your child needs to be free to assert his will, but he also needs to be able to move his bowels without discomfort. Celebrate every bowel movement that lands in the potty and don't make a fuss when training backslides, which happens now and then with almost every child.

Natural Remedies

All of the natural remedies listed below can be used to supplement conventional medical treatment.

Diet and Nutrition
For good food sources of particular nutrients, see pages 9–13.

- Lactobacillus acidophilus boosts the levels of beneficial bacteria in the intestine, which can help with digestion and relieve constipation. Give your child 1 dose a day, as directed on the product label.

Herbal
Use one or more of the remedies listed below. Dosage varies according to age; see the chart on page 25 to determine the correct dose for your child.

- Licorice tea soothes the intestines and helps relieve constipation. Give your child 1 dose of licorice tea twice a day for 3 or 4 days.
- Psyllium is Mother Nature's laxative (in addition to being the active ingredient in many over-the-counter laxative preparations). Give your child ½ teaspoon of psyllium seeds 3 times a day, or as directed on the package.

Homeopathy
Use one homeopathic treatment at a time, based on your child's specific symptoms. For dosage information, see the chart on pages 31–37. Discontinue use if the symptoms disappear.

- *Alumina* 30x or 9c: Use if your child's stools are small, hard, dry pellets, often covered with mucus. Give 1 dose 2 or 3 times daily for 2 or 3 days.
- *Lycopodium (Lycopodium clavatum)* 30x or 9c: Use if your child has hard, dry stools and experiences pain right before a bowel movement. Give 1 dose 2 or 3 times daily for 2 or 3 days.
- *Nux (Strychnos nux vomica)* 6c: Use if your child feels the urge to defecate but is unable to, or if he finishes and feels there is more to come. Give 1 dose 4 times daily for up to 14 days.

Acupressure

Use one or more of the acupressure points listed below. For a diagram showing the specific pressure points, see pages 40–41.

- Crooked Pond (Large Intestine 11): This point is located on the forearm at the outer edge of the elbow crease.
- Joining the Valley (Large Intestine 4): To find this point, place your fingers at the highest spot of the muscle on the back of the hand that protrudes when the thumb and index finger are pressing close together.
- Sea of Energy (Conception Vessel 6): Apply steady pressure on the point 3 child's finger widths directly below the belly button.
- Three Mile Point (Stomach 36): This point is located 4 child's finger widths below the kneecap, 1 child's finger width to the outside of the shinbone. If you are on the correct spot, a muscle should flex as you move your foot up and down.

An Ounce of Prevention

The best way to prevent constipation is to be sure your child drinks plenty of fluids, eats plenty of fiber, and gets plenty of exercise.

When to Call for Help

Constipation usually clears up without a doctor's intervention, but you should contact your pediatrician if your infant becomes constipated, or fails to have a bowel movement within 3 or 4 days, since the problem could indicate an intestinal blockage. With older children, call the doctor if there is blood in the stool, significant abdominal pain, or if your child has accidental bowel movements, in addition to constipation. If your child's constipation seems to be rooted in an emotional conflict or toilet training problem, talk to your doctor.

Cough

It starts with a tickle in the back of the throat, but there's nothing funny about a persistent and irrepressible urge to cough. Coughing is actually the body's way of clearing the lungs, and in most cases, you should leave your child alone and let him cough, especially if he is successful in bringing up mucus. Coughing also helps the lungs clear themselves of bacteria, dust, pollen, and other irritants.

Coughing can be caused by a bacterial or viral infection, a blockage in the airway, or even by breathing a lungful of uncomfortably hot or cold air. Of course, coughing should be controlled when the hacking keeps your child (and you) up all night. During the day, however, you should try to make your child as comfortable as possible, but let him cough it out.

Traditional Treatments

Tank up. Drinking clear fluids helps thin the mucus in the lungs, making it easier to cough up. Hot drinks can be very comforting and the moisture can soothe the throat and lungs, but any clear beverage or soup will do (especially chicken soup).

If it's an allergy . . . Antihistamines can be used at night to help your child sleep if the cough is caused by an allergic reaction, rather than a bacterial or viral infection. You can tell an allergic reaction is the culprit if the cough follows your child's exposure to trigger allergens. (For more information on allergies, see page 58.) Follow all package directions and dosage information to the letter.

In search of a good night's sleep. If your child hasn't slept in a couple of nights and the cough lingers on, consider a dose of over-the-counter cough suppressant before bedtime. Again, read and follow the package instructions for proper usage.

Natural Remedies

All of the natural remedies listed below can be used to supplement conventional medical treatment.

Diet and Nutrition

Use one or more of the remedies listed below. Dosage varies according to age; see the chart on pages 14–15 to determine to correct dose for your child. For good food sources of particular nutrients, see pages 9–13.

- Vitamin C helps reduce inflammation and strengthen the immune system. Give your child 1 dose of vitamin C 3 times a day.
- Zinc lozenges boost the immune system, fight infection, and reduce inflammation of the throat and lungs. Give your child 1 lozenge 2 or 3 times daily, as needed.

Herbal

Use one or more of the remedies listed below. Dosage varies according to age; see the chart on page 25 to determine the correct dose for your child.

- Both coltsfoot and licorice tea can help clear congestion from the lungs and soothe the respiratory tract. Give your child 1 dose of either tea 3 times daily for 2 or 3 days.

- Lungwort is an herb well-known as a cough remedy. Give your child 1 dose 3 times daily for 2 or 3 days.
- Mullein tea can relieve a cough, especially during the early stages of an illness. Give your child 1 dose 3 times daily for 2 days as soon as the coughing begins.

Homeopathy

Use one homeopathic treatment at a time, based on your child's specific symptoms. For dosage information, see the chart on pages 31–37. Discontinue use if the symptoms disappear.

- *Antimonium tart. (Antimonium tartaricum)* 30x or 9c: Use if your child feels breathless due to thick mucus. Give 1 dose 3 times daily for 2 days.
- *Belladonna (Atropha belladonna)* 30x or 9c: Use if your child has a fever with the cough. Give 1 dose 3 times daily for 1 day.
- *Pulsatilla (Pulsatilla nigricans)* 30x or 9c: Use if your child has a loose cough and yellowish nasal discharge. Give 1 dose 3 times daily for 2 days.
- *Spongia (Spongia tosta)* 12x or 6c: Use if your child has a dry barking cough. Give 1 dose 3 times daily for 2 days.

Acupressure

Use one or more of the acupressure points listed below. For a diagram showing the specific pressure points, see pages 40–41.

- Lung Associated Point (Bladder 13): This point is located 1 child's finger width below the upper tip of the shoulder blade, between the spine and the scapula.
- Vital Diaphragm (Bladder 38): To find this point, place your fingers between the shoulder blade and the spine at the level of the heart.
- Elegant Mansion (Kidney 27): Apply steady pressure on the point in the hollow below the collarbone next to the breastbone.
- Letting Go (Lung 1): This point is located on the outer part of the chest, 3 child's finger widths below the collarbone.

- Fish Border (Lung 10): To find this point, place your fingers on the palm side of your child's hand in the center of the pad at the base of the thumb.

An Ounce of Prevention

To prevent coughing, avoid exposing your child to other sick children. If your child has a respiratory allergy, try to avoid exposing your child to the trigger allergens.

When to Call for Help

Coughing has a number of causes, from the benign to the serious. It can be caused by a viral or bacterial infection, asthma, allergies, or a more serious condition, such as cystic fibrosis. If your child's cough lasts more than 1 week, if your child has difficulty breathing, or if your child comes down with a fever, contact your doctor.

Cradle Cap

Most parents cringe when they discover the telltale signs of cradle cap—yellow, crusty patches on an infant's scalp, face, armpits, or groin area—but the condition is not dangerous, and in most cases it doesn't bother the baby a bit.

Cradle cap (also known as *Seborrheic Eczema*) is caused by overproductive sebaceous (oil) glands. These glands work overtime and secrete excessive oil, which then dries and plugs the ducts, forming greasy, scaly patches. In attempting to un-plug the clog, the oil glands continue to pump out oil, and the unsightly "cap" becomes thicker and deeper.

The condition is most common in infants less than three months of age, but it can show up in older children, too. It usually disappears on its own, but you may want to take steps to hasten its departure.

Traditional Treatments

- *Go easy on the suds.* The more you wash your baby's hair, the more oil the sebaceous glands will produce. Wash every other day, but do a thorough job on the scrub days.
- *Get tough on grime.* If your doctor gives you the go-ahead, switch to an over-the-counter dandruff-fighting shampoo for use once or twice a week. The tingly formula may help loosen the scales, but it's powerful stuff, so be careful not to let it drip in baby's eyes. You may want to experiment with using a visor to shield your child's face while shampooing; some children tolerate them well, others find them disconcerting.
- *Follow your doctor's orders.* When cradle cap shows up behind your baby's ears or elsewhere on the face, neck, or in the diaper area, talk to your doctor about using a 0.5 percent hydrocortisone cream 2 or 3 times a day. The drug is available over-the-counter, but don't be lulled into believing that it's a mild medication. Talk to your doctor about the appropriate dosage.

Natural Remedies

All of the natural remedies listed below can be used to supplement conventional medical treatment.

Diet and Nutrition
Use one or more of the remedies listed below. Dosage varies according to age; see the chart on pages 14–15 to determine to correct dose for your child. Some vitamins can be used topically, as noted. For good food sources of particular nutrients, see pages 9–13.

- Nursing mothers should consider taking the supplement Lactobacillus acidophilus, which can help prevent fungal infec-

tions. Follow the dosage instructions on the label.
- Apply a vitamin B$_6$ salve to affected spots on your infant's scalp, twice daily, for 2 days.
- Before washing your child's hair, gently rub it with olive oil or vitamin E oil to loosen the flakes. Leave the oil on the hair for 15 minutes, then use a toothbrush to gently massage the scaly areas before washing thoroughly.

Herbal

- After washing your child's scalp, apply calendula ointment. Use a fine-tooth comb to brush away loose flakes.

Homeopathy

Use one homeopathic treatment at a time, based on your child's specific symptoms. For dosage information, see the chart on pages 31–37. Discontinue use if the symptoms disappear.

- *Graphites* 6c: Use if the crusted areas are weepy and easily infected. Give 1 dose every 4 hours, for up to 2 weeks.
- *Viola (Viola tricolor)* 6c: Use if the crusted areas are thick and patchy. Give 1 dose every 4 hours, for up to 2 weeks.

An Ounce of Prevention

Don't take it personally: Cradle cap can take hold even if you wash your baby's head and hair every day. You may be able to ward off some cases by keeping your child's scalp scrupulously clean and dry. Gently but firmly wash the scalp of excess oil; your baby's head may seem fragile, but it is tough enough to withstand a vigorous washing.

When to Call for Help

When shampooing your baby's hair, look for signs of infection. If you see any pus, or if the area is tender and red, see your doctor or pediatrician. An infection can easily be treated with oral antibiotics. Also contact your doctor if the cradle cap does not respond to treatment within 6 weeks; it could be a sign of a more serious skin problem.

Croup

When it comes to croup, its bark is worse than its bite. Croup is a viral infection of the vocal cords characterized by a hoarse, barking cough that usually appears in the middle of the night. The illness is frightening, but usually benign.

Croup usually strikes children between 3 months and 4 years of age because their airways are narrower and clog with mucus more easily than those of adults. It isn't caused by a particular virus, but instead is a symptom of a number of different viruses. Croup often follows a sore throat, cold, or laryngitis.

The illness typically starts with a case of the sniffles and a low fever. After several days of these mild symptoms, your child awakens in the night with the classic cough that sounds like a seal barking. At this stage, the voice box and windpipe have become inflamed. This swelling may make it somewhat difficult for your child to breathe. Some children also emit a vibrating sound when they inhale (known as a stridor).

Traditional Treatments

- *Take a deep breath.* The more relaxed and calm you are, the easier it will be for your child to feel relaxed and calm. The more anxious your child feels, the worse his symptoms will be.
- *First, try hot water.* Many parents find that warm steam eases their children's breathing, perhaps because it decreases the swelling in the airway. Sit with your child in the bath-

room while a hot shower runs for 15 or 20 minutes. The steamier, the better.

- *Then, try cold air.* Cool night air opens airways for some children with croup. (Many embarrassed parents have bundled their gasping children into their cars and rushed to the emergency room, only to find their children breathing normally by the time they arrive.) Dress your child appropriately and try taking him out into the cool night air, either for a walk or a drive. If you don't want to leave home, try sitting next to an open window. Or, if you live in a warm area, try cranking up the air conditioning to see if your child's symptoms are relieved.
- *Drink up.* The combination of fever and heavy breathing can cause your child to become dehydrated. Offer your child plenty of fluids.
- *Listen carefully.* For your child's comfort—and for your own—consider sleeping in your child's room (or bringing him into your room) for the night. You want to be available to console your child and to monitor him throughout the night to make sure his condition does not become worse. Croup tends to become much worse at night, so snuggle in and try to get some rest.

Natural Remedies

All of the natural remedies listed below can be used to supplement conventional medical treatment.

Diet and Nutrition

Use one or more of the remedies listed below. Dosage varies according to age; see the chart on pages 14–15 to determine to correct dose for your child. For good food sources of particular nutrients, see pages 9–13.

- Have your child drink plenty of fluids. Staying well hydrated will help thin mucus secretions and make coughing more productive.
- Vitamin C can boost the immune system and help fight in-

fection. Give your child 1 dose of vitamin C 3 times a day
for 3 days.

Herbal

Dosage varies according to age; see the chart on page 25 to
determine the correct dose for your child.

- Offer your child chamomile tea to soothe and relax him.

Homeopathy

Use one homeopathic treatment at a time, based on your
child's specific symptoms. For dosage information, see the
chart on pages 31–37. Discontinue use if the symptoms disappear.

- *Aconite (Aconitum napellus)* 6x or 12x: Use if your child is
  restless with a loud, dry cough. Give 1 dose at onset of
  illness and a second an hour later.
- *Ferrum phos. (Ferrum phosphoricum)* 12x or 6c: Use if your
  child has croup and a fever. Give 1 dose every 4 hours for
  up to 3 doses.
- *Kali mur. (Kali muriaticum)* 12x or 6c: Use if your child
  has croup. Give 1 dose every 4 hours for the first 3 doses;
  then give 1 dose 3 times daily for 2 days.

Acupressure

Use one or more of the acupressure points listed below. For
a diagram showing the specific pressure points, see pages 40–
41.

- Inner Gate (Pericardium 6): This point is located in the center of the inner forearm 2½ child's finger widths from the
  wrist crease.
- Sea of Tranquility (Conception Vessel 17): To find this
  point, put your fingers on the center of the breastbone, 3
  child's thumb widths up from the base of the bone.

An Ounce of Prevention

There's little you can do to prevent croup, aside from trying to keep your child healthy and well rested—and keeping your fingers crossed.

When to Call for Help

One problem with croup is that it can be confused with two other serious illnesses—epiglottis (inflammation of the cartilage flap at the top of the throat) and infectious tracheitis (inflammation of the windpipe caused by a staph infection). Both of these diseases can be life-threatening if the swelling blocks the windpipe; both are usually accompanied by a fever. If you suspect either condition rather than simple croup, call your doctor or get to the emergency room as soon as possible. WARNING: Do not open your child's mouth to look inside and assess the swelling. This can block your child's airway.

When you're dealing with run-of-the-mill croup, most cases aren't serious and can be handled at home. Of course, if you are worried about your child's breathing—or just need some reassurance—you should call your doctor. In addition, call your doctor if your child has a fever of 103 degrees F or higher, excessive drooling, labored breathing, pale color, or if your child cannot bend his neck forward.

Cuts, Scrapes, and Scratches

Accidents happen, though they do seem to happen to some kids more than others. Cuts, scrapes, and scratches are part of being a kid: Falls, bumps, and slips can't be avoided when you're learning to walk, climb stairs, ride a bike, and how to be a big kid. Some cuts, scrapes, and scratches can be cured with a reassuring hug and a kiss-to-make-it-better, but others require more extensive treatment (in addition to the hugs and kisses).

Cuts, scrapes, and scratches require different treatment. Cuts slice into the skin, and scrapes and scratches involve damage to the surface of the skin. The deeper and more extensive the injury, the greater the need for medical help. If an injury is deep enough for the skin to remain gaping open, it may require stitches and should be seen by a doctor. However, most simple injuries involve only the skin and the layer of fatty tissue just beneath the skin, and they can be treated at home. More serious injuries to the underlying muscles, tendons, ligaments, and nerves demand professional medical treatment and run the risk of causing long-lasting damage.

Traditional Treatments

Put the pressure on. To stop the bleeding, especially with a cut or scrape, cover the injury with a clean cloth and apply pressure directly to the wound. (If you don't have a clean rag, use your clothing, or apply your hand directly.) Apply firm pressure for 5–10 minutes.

Clean it up. Once the bleeding has stopped, the wound should be cleaned thoroughly with soap and water; hydrogen peroxide can be used as well. If you leave bits of dirt or gravel in a scrape, they can remain in the wound and cause scarring, in addition to increasing the risk of infection. (Extensive scrapes with deeply embedded dirt should be cleaned out by a medical professional, who may need to use a local anesthetic to calm your child during the cleaning.) When the wound is clean, apply an antibacterial cream or ointment to reduce the risk of infection.

To cover or not to cover? For cuts, cover the injury with a bandage or sterile gauze pad. For scrapes, leave the area uncovered and exposed to air and sunlight to help the body form Mother Nature's bandage, a scab. If the scrape is apt to get dirty when your child plays outside, cover it with a loose bandage during play, then rewash the area and leave it uncovered when your child comes in at the end of the day.

Wait. Leave the wound alone for 1–2 days. No peeking

under the bandage. The wound needs at least this long to begin healing, and frequent examination will interfere with the process.

Need a shot in the arm? Check your child's medical records to be sure his tetanus vaccination is up to date. Tetanus is included in the series of childhood vaccinations, but booster shots are required every 10 years to maintain immunity. If your child needs a booster shot, call your doctor.

Natural Remedies

All of the natural remedies listed below can be used to supplement conventional medical treatment.

Diet and Nutrition

Use one or more of the remedies listed below. Dosage varies according to age; see the chart on pages 14–15 to determine to correct dose for your child. Some vitamins can be used topically, as noted. For good food sources of particular nutrients, see pages 9–13.

- Vitamin C with bioflavonoids helps heal the skin and boost the immune system. Give your child 1 dose 2 or 3 times a day for 5 days.
- Vitamin E helps heal the skin when taken internally, and prevent scarring when used externally. Give your child 1 dose of vitamin E daily for 5 days. Apply vitamin E oil directly to a cut after a scab has formed to minimize scarring.

Herbal

Use one or more of the topical remedies listed below.

- Aloe vera gel soothes the skin and speeds healing. Apply fresh gel directly to the wound after cleaning.
- Calendula ointment helps kill bacteria and speed the healing process. Apply the ointment to the wound after cleaning.

Homeopathy

Use one homeopathic treatment at a time, based on your child's specific symptoms. For dosage information, see the chart on page 25. Discontinue use if the symptoms disappear.

- *Arnica (Arnica montana)* 30c: Use if your child's cut is deep and requires stitching. Give 1 dose after the stitches and repeat every 30 minutes for up to 6 doses.
- *Staphisagria (Delphinium staphisagria)* 6c: Use if your child's wound is very painful. Give 1 dose every 6 hours for up to 3 days.

An Ounce of Prevention

You can't prevent your child from being exposed to many of life's unpleasantries, but you can keep an eye out for obvious dangers and forbid your child from engaging in stupid, hazardous activities. But a good many falls and tumbles will happen despite your efforts, so just try to be on hand to comfort—and clean up the cuts, scrapes, and scratches.

When to Call for Help

If a cut is deep or wide enough to cause the skin to gape open, it probably needs a stitch or two to help with the healing (if you just let the wound heal on its own, the resulting scar will be much bigger than if the wound is sutured). If this type of wound is on the face, you'll want to ask for a plastic surgeon so that there will be minimal risk of permanent scarring. Act promptly: If you wait more than 8 hours, your doctor may not want to close the wound because of the increased risk of bacterial infection in a wound that has been open that long.

Cuts deep enough to cut a tendon or ligament, or those that won't stop bleeding, should be considered medical emergencies; get to a hospital emergency room immediately.

Redness around the edges of a wound are part of the healing process, but more extensive redness, in addition to swelling, fever, and pus or discharge, indicate that the wound has become infected. Don't worry about the clear fluid or serum weeping from scrapes: The clear fluid helps form the scab, but thick, yellow pus is a sign of infection. The signs of infection won't show up for at least 24 hours, until the bacteria have a chance to multiply. If you notice a problem after that, contact your doctor, who can and probably will prescribe antibiotics.

Dandruff

Dandruff can be extremely difficult to live with. It's not that the problem itself is anything to be worried about, or is difficult to treat, but the other kids at school can be downright cruel.

Explain to your child that the telltale white flakes of dandruff are nothing more than excess skin. Everybody has dandruff to some degree because every body is constantly shedding skin cells and growing new ones. And dandruff is nothing unusual: As many as 1 in 5 people has a scalp that sheds enough skin cells to have them show up as white flakes or scales.

When your child protests: Why me? Tell him you don't know. Researchers aren't sure either. Some think dandruff is caused by a microscopic fungus on the scalp, but others think it has more to do with the rapid production of new skin cells. What researchers do know is that dandruff doesn't hurt the hair, it doesn't cause baldness, and it doesn't mean the hair is necessarily greasy or unclean.

Traditional Treatments

- *Lather up.* Buy an over-the-counter dandruff shampoo and have your child give it a try. Start by having your child use the product at least twice a week, and if that doesn't work shampoo more often with your regular shampoo. Blondes beware: Products containing tar can stain lighter hair, so check the list of ingredients.

- *Take your time.* It takes time for the medicated shampoos to work effectively on the scalp. Follow the package instructions; many products recommend leaving the lather on the hair for 5 minutes before rinsing. Many products suggest you lather twice—once to remove the flakes and a second time to treat the scalp.
- *Easy on the oil.* If you have a teenager who uses hair styling products, suggest she use oil-free products. Greasy conditioners, mousses, and other treatments will make the problem worse.
- *Easy come, easy go.* It will take work to keep your child's scalp flake-free. Once the problem is under control, switch back to your regular shampoo, but keep the antidandruff formula in the medicine cabinet. You may need to use it again before long.

Natural Remedies

All of the natural remedies listed below can be used to supplement conventional medical treatment.

Herbal
Use one or more of the remedies listed below.

- Massage the scalp with olive and rosemary oil. Leave the oil on the hair for 20 minutes, then brush out the loose flakes and shampoo.
- Thyme has antiseptic properties that can help alleviate dandruff. Boil 2 tablespoons of dried thyme in 1 cup of water for 10 minutes. Strain, cool, and pour water through clean, damp hair. Massage the mixture into the scalp. Do not rinse.
- To ease the itch, apply calendula ointment to irritated areas around the hairline.

Homeopathy

Use one homeopathic treatment at a time, based on your child's specific symptoms. For dosage information, see the chart on pages 31–37. Discontinue use if the symptoms disappear.

- *Arsenicum (Arsenicum album)* 6c: Use if your child's scalp is dry, hot, and itchy at night. Give 1 dose 3 times daily for 1 week.
- *Sepia (Sepia officinalis)* 6c: Use if your child's scalp is moist, greasy, and sensitive around hair roots. Give 1 dose 3 times daily for 1 week.
- *Sulphur* 6c: Use if your child's dandruff is thick and burning. Give 3 times a day for 1 week.

An Ounce of Prevention

Wash your child's hair often with nondrying shampoos, such as products designed for infants and children, or those with conditioners. If your child uses hair-styling products, encourage the use of those that do not contain alcohol to avoid drying the scalp further.

When to Call for Help

Check with your doctor if your child's dandruff persists after 2 weeks of home treatment. Don't wait that long if you notice hair loss, or if your child complains that his scalp is painful, inflamed, or really itchy. Other skin problems, such as ringworm and other fungal infections, can look a bit like dandruff, even though they require different treatment.

Diaper Rash

There's no use feeling guilty: Chances are good that your baby will develop diaper rash sometime in his young life, no matter how diligent you are about changing him at the first sign (or smell) of trouble.

Diaper rash is the result of your baby's sensitive skin sharing cramped quarters with the toxic combination of acidic urine and feces. The noxious mixture breaks down the protective oils on baby's bottom, leaving a red, swollen, sore area behind.

Diaper rash can occur in babies of any age, but the most common problem time is around 9 months. Experimenting with new foods can trigger an outbreak, as can dehydration, diarrhea, and use of antibiotics.

In most cases, the rash disappears in a day or so, but the irritation can linger on for 10 days or more. Though every parent tends to have a strong preference for either cloth or disposable diapers for a number of reasons, there is evidence the superabsorbent disposables keep baby's skin drier and closer to normal pH than cloth diapers or regular disposables.

Traditional Treatments

- *The more air the better.* The easiest way to treat the problem is to let your baby spend as much time as possible out of diapers. Let your baby roam diaper-free in a warm, dry room. The rash almost always clears up when exposed to air. Just 10 or 15 minutes after a diaper change should be enough to do the trick.
- *Change is good.* Especially when you're changing diapers. The sooner you change your little one's dirty diaper, the fresher his bottom will be.

- *Build a barrier.* Apply Desitin or another zinc oxide ointment to the diaper area to heal the rash and dry the sores. The ointment forms a protective layer between your baby's delicate skin and those harsh, nasty chemicals. The ointment can be drying, so don't use it if your baby's skin is dry or scaly.
- *Eliminate the breeding ground.* Throw out the plastic pants. If your little one wears cloth diapers, use cloth diaper covers. The plastic traps the moisture and creates an ideal environment for the spread of the rash. If your child wears disposable diapers, put them on loose enough to allow for a little air circulation, at least until the rash clears.
- *Be a water baby.* Soaking in a warm bath for 5 or 10 minutes a couple of times a day can go a long way toward soothing your baby's bottom. The water will remove the irritating acids, restore moisture and promote healing.
- *Pass on the alcohol.* Many commercial baby wipes contain alcohol, perfume and other chemicals that can bother baby's bottom, especially during an outbreak of diaper rash. Though many parents rely on the convenience of diaper wipes, switch to mild soap and water and thoroughly rinse, at least until the rash has passed.

Natural Remedies

All of the natural remedies listed below can be used to supplement conventional medical treatment.

Diet and Nutrition

Use one or more of the remedies listed below. Dosage varies according to age; see the chart on pages 14–15 to determine to correct dose for your child. Some vitamins can be used topically, as noted. For good food sources of particular nutrients, see pages 9–13.

- Make sure your baby is getting plenty of fluids to dilute the powerful acids present in urine and feces.
- Closely monitor the introduction of new foods into your baby's diet. Many parents associate diaper rash with the intro-

duction of new foods. If you suspect a particular food is the culprit, remove it from your child's diet and try again a few weeks later.

- Lactobacillus acidophilus supplements and helps encourage the growth of "good" bacteria that keep the body healthy. Nursing mothers can take the dose listed on the package. Bottle-fed infants can get ⅛ teaspoon mixed with formula once a day for up to a week.
- If the diaper area is very dry and irritated, rub some vitamin E oil into the irritated skin at changing time.

Herbal

- Apply a thin coating of calendula ointment after a diaper change.

Homeopathy

Use one homeopathic treatment at a time, based on your child's specific symptoms. For dosage information, see the chart on pages 31–37. Discontinue use if the symptoms disappear.

- *Rhus tox. (Rhus toxicodendron)* 6c: Use if the skin is itchy, with little blisters. Give 1 dose 4 times daily for up to 5 days.
- *Sulphur* 6c: Use if the rash is dry, red and scaly. Give 1 dose twice daily for up to 3 days.

Acupressure

For a diagram showing the specific pressure point, see pages 40–41.

- Bigger Rushing (Liver 3): This point is located on the top of the foot in the valley between the big toe and the second toe.

An Ounce of Prevention

The best way to prevent diaper rash is to change your baby as soon as he wets or soils his diaper. Clean the area well, particularly between skin folds. If your baby develops frequent diaper rashes, sponge the area affected by the diaper rash with a mixture of 1 tablespoon of baking soda and 4 ounces of water. The alkalinity of baking soda should help to counterbalance the acidity of urine and stool.

When to Call for Help

Most diaper rashes disappear in a day or two, but some robust rashes last more than a week, long enough to merit a call to the doctor. Look for signs of infection—fever, loss of appetite, swelling, discharge, pimple-like blisters—and contact your doctor, who may prescribe an antibiotic.

Diarrhea

The digestive system isn't very discriminating. When confronted with a toxin, the system shifts into overdrive and simply clears itself of anything—and everything—in the way. The result, diarrhea, involves frequent, loose or watery stools and abdominal cramping.

Diarrhea can be caused by viruses, bacteria, protozoa, food poisoning, food allergy, lactose intolerance, or dietary imbalance, such as too much fiber. The condition is not only unpleasant, it can be dangerous if the fluids lost by the body are not replenished in a timely fashion. Most bouts of diarrhea clear up within 24 hours, but the potentially life-threatening complications of dehydration can show up in a matter of hours in a small child, so it demands immediate attention and treatment.

Traditional Treatments

Drink up. The immediate risk of diarrhea is dehydration, and the best way to prevent it is to encourage your child to drink as frequently as possible. Try water, crushed ice, ginger ale, or oral rehydration treatments. Give your child as much fluid as possible. Infants less than 20 pounds should receive 3 ounces of liquid per pound per day to avoid dehydration; babies over 20 pounds should get 1½ ounces per pound per day.

Don't force the feeding. When your child is ready for chow, he'll ask for it. Start feeding with the BRAT diet—bananas, rice, applesauce, and toast—because these foods help with stool formation. Some parents swear that strained carrots will clear the situation in no time. If your child asks for a particular food, give it a try; most kids know what their stomachs can handle. One exception: Avoid milk and dairy products, which can be hard to digest during illness.

Hold the apple juice. Too much of a good thing can cause diarrhea. Fruit juice, particularly apple juice, can loosen the stools. Limit the juice to 2 half-cup servings a day. If your little one craves more, dilute the allotted amount with water.

Switch to sugar. Skip foods and beverages containing artificial sweeteners, such as sorbitol and saccharin, which can promote diarrhea.

Talk to your doctor before you head to the drugstore. Yes, the pharmacy shelves are stocked with over-the-counter treatments for diarrhea, but many physicians do not recommend their use. Talk to your doctor before dosing your child.

Natural Remedies

All of the natural remedies listed below can be used to supplement conventional medical treatment.

Diet and Nutrition

- Lactobacillus acidophilus restores beneficial bacteria to the intestinal tract. Give your child 1 dose twice a day for 5–7 days, following dosage information on the label.

Herbal

- Goldenseal helps overcome intestinal distress caused by bacterial infections. Give your child 5 drops twice a day for 1 or 2 days. Do not administer to a child under age 4.

Homeopathy

Use one homeopathic treatment at a time, based on your child's specific symptoms. For dosage information, see the chart on pages 31–37. Discontinue use if the symptoms disappear. If diarrhea continues after 1 or 2 days, contact your pediatrician.

- *Arsenicum (Arsenicum album)* 30x or 9c: Use if your child's diarrhea appears to be related to food poisoning, anxiety, or stress, rather than a viral infection. Give 1 dose 3 or 4 times daily, for 1 or 2 days.
- *Calcarea (Calcarea carbonica)* 30x or 9c: Use if your child develops diarrhea after eating dairy products. Give 1 dose 3–4 times a day, for 1 or 2 days.
- *Magnesia phos. (Magnesia phosphorica)* 12x or 6c: Use if your child is experiencing cramping in addition to diarrhea. Give 1 dose 3–4 times daily, for 1 or 2 days.
- *Pulsatilla (Pulsatilla nigricans)* 30x or 9c: Use if your child has diarrhea after eating fatty foods, especially at night. Give 1 dose 3–4 times a day, for 1 or 2 days.

Acupressure

Use one or more of the acupressure points listed below. For a diagram showing the specific pressure points, see pages 40–41.

- Abdominal Sorrow (Spleen 16): This point is located below the edge of the rib cage a ½ inch inside the nipple line.

- Grandfather Grandson (Spleen 4): To find this point, place your fingers on the arch of the foot, 1 child's thumb width in back of the ball of the foot.
- Sea of Energy (Conception Vessel 6): Apply steady pressure on the point 2 child's finger widths directly below the belly button.
- Travel Between (Liver 2): This point is located at the juncture of the big and second toes.

An Ounce of Prevention

Meticulous hand-washing habits may prevent some outbreaks of diarrhea caused by food poisoning or bacterial infection. If you suspect a food allergy or lactose intolerance due to recurring diarrhea after eating certain foods, monitor your child's diet carefully (see page 58 for more information).

When to Call for Help

With diarrhea, you need to look out for signs of dehydration. Symptoms include: infrequent urination, dark or concentrated urine, crying without tears, loss of skin elasticity, and lethargy. In infants, also look for a sunken fontanelle, the "soft spot" at the top of the baby's head. Call your doctor if your child experiences both diarrhea and vomiting, which increases the possibility of dehydration. In addition, contact your doctor immediately if your child experiences bloody diarrhea, severe abdominal cramping, or if the diarrhea persists for more than 2 or 3 days.

Dizziness

Dizziness is disturbing to adults and can be downright frightening to small children who don't understand what is going on when they feel that the room is spinning, or that the floor is tipping over to one side.

At the most basic level, dizziness involves an insufficient oxygen supply to the brain, which results in a false feeling or perception of movement. Dizziness is usually accompanied by nausea, cold sweats, and a lack of depth perception. It can be caused by heat, poor ventilation, motion sickness, a virus, or low blood sugar in the afternoon after your child has skipped lunch. Other times dizziness stems from an infection of the inner ear, which maintains and controls the body's perception of balance.

Traditional Treatments

Lie down. The first thing to do when your child feels dizzy is to have him slowly lie down and relax. Lying flat will allow the blood to circulate to the head, in addition to eliminating any risk of injury due to falling. Another option is to have him sit in a chair and rest his head between his knees to increase blood circulation to the brain.

The after-bath blues. If your little one feels like he's spinning after soaking in a steamy tub for a half hour or so, have him sip a cool drink and lie down. The hot tub has caused the blood to rush to the surface of the skin, diminishing the blood flow to the brain. A few minutes of cooling off and the dizziness will pass.

Eat, drink, and be steady. Dehydration and low blood sugar levels can cause dizziness in children who do not eat and drink frequently enough during the day. Encourage your child to eat

148

regular meals and to snack, if needed, to keep energy levels up during play.

Get into focus. Little kids love to do somersaults and to spin around in circles until they collapse in a giggling heap on the grass. This kind of play can lead to a serious case of the dizzies. If your child spins himself silly, have him focus on a nearby stationary object (such as his foot or shoe) to help settle his inner ear and help him regain his bearings and sense of balance.

Natural Remedies

All of the natural remedies listed below can be used to supplement conventional medical treatment.

Diet and Nutrition

- If you suspect low blood sugar is the source of the problem because your child has not eaten in 4 or 5 hours, give him a glass of fruit juice (any kind) to boost his sugar level immediately.

Herbal

Use one or more of the remedies listed below. Dosage varies according to age; see the chart on page 25 to determine the correct dose for your child.

- Ginger relieves both nausea and dizziness. Give your child either 1 dose of ginger tea or a dose of ginger in capsule form.
- You may be able to clear your child's head by giving him a whiff of herbal smelling salts made with rosemary oil or peppermint oil. Put 4 or 5 drops of the oil on a clean cloth and have your child inhale a deep breath with the cloth almost touching his nose.

Homeopathy

Use one homeopathic treatment at a time, based on your child's specific symptoms. For dosage information, see the chart on pages 31–37. Discontinue use if the symptoms disappear.

- *Calcarea (Calcarea carbonica)* 6c: Use if dizziness becomes worse when looking up. Give 1 dose as often as necessary for up to 10 doses.
- *Conium (Conium maculatum)* 6c: Use if dizziness becomes worse when lying down. Give 1 dose as often as necessary for up to 10 doses.
- *Gelsemium (Gelsemium sempervirens)* 6c: Use if your child feels trembly as well as dizzy. Give 1 dose as often as necessary for up to 10 doses.
- *Nux (Strychnos nux vomica)* 6c: Use if dizziness becomes worse around flickering lights. Give 1 dose as often as necessary for up to 10 doses.

Acupressure

Use one or more of the acupressure points listed below. For a diagram showing the specific pressure points, see pages 40–41.

- Gates of Consciousness (Gallbladder 20): This point is located just below the base of the skull, outside the hollow between the two large neck muscles.
- Middle of a Person (Governing Vessel 26): To find this point, place your fingers ⅔ of the way up from the upper lip to the nose.
- Sea of Energy (Conception Vessel 6): Apply steady pressure on the point 3 child's finger widths below the belly button.
- Sea of Vitality (Bladder 23 and Bladder 47): This point is located in the lower back, between the second and third lumbar vertebrae, 2–4 child's finger widths away from the spine at waist level.

An Ounce of Prevention

Your child's dizziness may be caused by low blood sugar if the room starts spinning after your child has gone 4 or 5 hours without eating. Also, if your child eats a meal high in simple sugars, he may "crash" and experience low blood sugar levels two hours or so after overdoing the sweets. If your child has a problem with dizziness caused by low blood sugar, encourage him to eat smaller, more frequent meals. A diet rich in B complex vitamins and protein can also stave off diet-related dizziness.

Any easy way to prevent dizziness caused by reading in the car: Slip in a bookmark and stop reading. For information on dizziness caused by inner ear infections, see below.

When to Call for Help

A bout of dizziness that passes within an hour or so isn't cause for alarm, unless it becomes a recurring problem. However, severe or long-lasting dizziness or dizziness that leads to fainting should be brought to your pediatrician's attention. Dizziness following a blow to the head demands immediate medical care.

Earache and Ear Infection

To some degree, it's the luck of the draw. Some kids constantly suffer from earaches and ear infections, and others get through childhood with nary a one. One reason may be differences in the structure of the ear itself.

Your child's ear has three parts: The outer ear (where the sound waves are caught and directed into the ear canal toward the eardrum), the middle ear (where the sound waves vibrate and bounce around three tiny bones), and the inner ear (where a tiny spiral structure turns the vibrations into nerve impulses to the brain).

Many ear problems center around the eustachian tube, a small tube that connects the middle ear and the throat to equalize air pressure and avoid rupturing the eardrum. Unfortunately, the eustachian tube can also allow bacteria to travel from the throat and nose into the middle ear. Kids with shorter eustachian tubes tend to develop more ear infections than other kids because it's easier for the bacteria to invade the middle ear. When the eustachian tube becomes infected and inflamed, fluid builds up in the middle ear, decreasing hearing and causing a stuffy feeling in the head. As kids grow, the angle of the eustachian tubes changes, allowing fluids to drain more readily. That's why most of the ten million children who get ear infections each year are between the ages of 6 months and 3 years.

Alas, infections aren't the exclusive domain of the middle ear. Swimmer's ear is an infection of the outer ear that usually occurs in the summer when people are in the water a lot (though it can afflict nonswimmers as well). The infection shows up as itching or tingling outside the ear, sometimes with a yellowish discharge. If your child's ear hurts when you gently pull it and wiggle it, chances are good your child has an outer-ear infection and should see the doctor.

Traditional Treatments

Go for the flow. Drink plenty of fluids and run a humidifier or vaporizer in your child's bedroom to keep the mucus secretions as thin as possible (the thinner the mucus, the less likely it will clog the eustachian tube). If your child has a lot of nasal secretions, give him over-the-counter decongestants or nose drops to shrink the nasal membranes and open the eustachian tube.

No pain, your gain. Control the pain associated with an ear infection by giving your child acetaminophen. Your child should feel better 12–24 hours after taking an antibiotic, but you may need to give him a dose or 2 of painkiller until the antibiotic kicks in. Never give your child under age 18 aspirin (including "baby aspirin"), due to the possibility of contracting Reye's syndrome, a potentially fatal disorder of the brain and liver.

Clear away the ear wax. In most cases, ear wax won't bother you if you don't bother it. The wax (cerumen) waterproofs, protects, and cleans the ear canal by trapping dust and bacteria, and it contains enzymes that kill harmful bacteria. Problems can occur when the wax builds up, inhibiting hearing by interfering with the vibration of the eardrum.

To remove packed-down ear wax, put a few drops of olive oil or glycerine in the ear to loosen the wax, then gently flush the ear canal with a syringe (available at drugstores). If you use an over-the-counter ear wax preparation, follow the directions explicitly to avoid irritation. And heed the warnings against using cotton swabs; they only push the wax further into the ear canal and disrupt the little hairs inside the ears that help push foreign substances out of the ears.

Try a warm water bottle. Many kids find a hot-water bottle—filled with warm water, not hot—very soothing when used as a pillow or headrest. Wrap the bottle in a soft towel before having your child lie down on it.

Sleep standing up. Not quite, but you may find that your child feels better if the head of the bed or crib is raised so that the ears drain more naturally. Ear pain usually peaks at night when your child lies down because the tubes no longer drain as readily. Try a new angle and see if it provides relief.

Natural Remedies

All of the natural remedies listed below can be used to supplement conventional medical treatment.

Diet and Nutrition

Use one or more of the remedies listed below. Dosage varies according to age; see the chart on pages 14–15 to determine to correct dose for your child. For good food sources of particular nutrients, see pages 9–13.

- Lactobacillus acidophilus kills infectious bacteria and helps maintain beneficial bacteria in the intestine, which will be destroyed in children taking antibiotics to treat an ear infection. Give your child 1 dose a day for 1 week after taking an antibiotic, following package directions.
- Vitamin C and bioflavonoids help reduce inflammation associated with an ear infection. Give your child 1 dose 3 times daily for 1 week.

Herbal

Use one or more of the remedies listed below. Dosage varies according to age; see the chart on page 25 to determine the correct dose for your child.

- Echinacea kills bacteria and boosts the immune system. Give your child 1 dose 3 times a day for 3 days, followed by 1 dose a day for 4 more days.
- Garlic helps kill the bacteria associated with ear infections. Give your child 1 dose of odorless garlic a day for 5 days, or follow package directions.

Homeopathy

Use one homeopathic treatment at a time, based on your child's specific symptoms. For dosage information, see the chart on pages 31–37. Discontinue use if the symptoms disappear.

- *Belladonna (Atropha belladonna)* 30c: Use if your child experiences throbbing pain made worse by warmth. Give 1 dose every ½ hour for up to 6 doses.
- *Hepar sulph. (Hepar sulphuris calcareum)* 6c: Use if your child experiences throbbing pain, which is soothed by warmth. Give 1 dose every ½ hour for up to 6 doses.
- *Pulsatilla (Pulsatilla nigricans)* 6c: Use if your child feels pressure behind the eardrum that feels as if it is pushing outward. Give 1 dose every ½ hour, for up to 6 doses.

Acupressure

Use one or more of the acupressure points listed below. For a diagram showing the specific pressure points, see pages 40–41.

- Bigger Stream (Kidney 3): This point is located midway between the inside of the anklebone and the Achilles tendon in the back of the ankle.
- Listening Place (Small Intestine 19): To find this point, place your fingers directly in front of the ear opening in the depression that deepens when the mouth is open.
- Wind Screen (Triple Warmer 17): Apply steady pressure on the point in the indentation behind the earlobe.

An Ounce of Prevention

Some, but not all, ear infections can be prevented. You can reduce the likelihood of your child developing an ear problem by breast-feeding your infant for 6 months or longer (antibodies in the breast milk help ward off infections), and by holding your child in an upright position when bottle-feeding to prevent milk from flowing into the eustachian tube where it can cause infection.

A number of factors must be taken into consideration when making child care arrangements, but if your child is prone to ear infections, he may be better off at home with a baby-sitter rather than in day care with more kids (and more germs). And at home, you can cut down on the number of ear infections by keeping your home smoke-free; several studies show children of smokers have more ear infections than children of nonsmokers.

Children who develop frequent outer-ear infections may benefit from a 30-second after-bath ritual—blowing dry their ears. Outer-ear infections or swimmer's ear is caused by moisture in the outer ear, and keeping the ears bone-dry can help prevent infection. After bathing, hold a hair dryer 18 inches or so away from your child's ear and blow warm air into the ear. It should take only a minute or so to dry up any remaining moisture.

When to Call for Help

Ear infections often follow a cold or upper respiratory infection, so it can be hard to tell where the cold leaves off and the ear infection begins. If your child complains of ear pain, pulls on his ears, experiences any loss of hearing, or suffers from a fever, call your pediatrician, who may prescribe antibiotics.

If your child doesn't improve 24–48 hours after taking antibiotics, call again; a stronger antibiotic may be needed. In rare cases, recurrent ear infections can be caused by a milk allergy; talk to your doctor about this possibility if your child is under the age of 1 and experiences chronic ear infections.

If your child wakes up and there is a crusty yellowish or bloody discharge on the pillow, call the doctor. Your child may have a ruptured eardrum, especially if he had been complaining about ear pain. The eardrum will heal (in fact, the rupture is part of the body's healing process), but the doctor will probably want to prescribe antibiotics to speed the healing and prevent infection.

Eczema

Eczema is the skin's way of telling to you there's a problem. Those red, itchy patches announce to the world that your child suffers from dry skin caused by an allergy or local irritation. When your child persistently scratches the area, the skin gets thick, scaly and rough; sometimes the skin oozes and becomes crusty.

Eczema (*atopic* or *contact dermatitis*) can appear at any age, but it often shows up in babies less than 18 months of age. The condition usually disappears by the time the child reaches preschool age. It tends to be triggered by common allergies, such as hay fever, asthma, sensitivity to perfumes, chemical reactions, and food allergies. There appears to be a genetic link involving eczema: Children with eczema live in families with other eczema sufferers.

The condition is unpredictable and can strike any part of the body, but most outbreaks occur on the creases of the elbows and knees, behind the ears, and on the face and wrists.

Traditional Treatments

- *Did you take a bath?* In this case, you may hope the answer is "no." Daily baths and showers can dry skin and make eczema worse. Try a sponge bath every other day, and on bath days, try to keep tub time to a minimum. Use a bath gel or soap substitute that will clean the skin without drying. And choose a fragrance-free product; sometimes it's the perfume that triggers an outbreak.
- *Turn down the heat.* Soaking in a hot bath may feel good, but it removes oils from the skin. Give your child a lukewarm bath.
- *Don't rub-a-dub-dub.* Easy does it when washing skin affected by eczema. Harshly scrubbing the area will dry it further and make the condition worse. If possible, just rinse the area with warm water and a mild soap substitute. After your child steps out of the tub, slather on moisturizer to hold moisture in the skin.
- *If it itches, don't scratch.* Try to help your child resist the temptation to scratch the itchy area by keeping nails short. In small children, consider putting socks over the hands at night (older children will yank the socks off during the night).
- *Rinse, rinse, rinse.* Detergent residues can irritate delicate skin, so put your child's laundry through a double rinse cycle. Skip the fabric softener and dryer sheets, which also leave chemical traces behind.
- *Do something to stop the itching!* Give your child an anti-itching antihistamine to relieve the almost insatiable urge to scratch. (Follow package directions for dosage information.) To relieve the itch, you can also try an over-the-counter hydrocortisone ointment on the irritated areas.

Natural Remedies

All of the natural remedies listed below can be used to supplement conventional medical treatment.

Diet and Nutrition

Use one or more of the remedies listed below. Dosage varies according to age; see the chart on pages 14–15 to determine to correct dose for your child. Some vitamins can be used topically, as noted. For good food sources of particular nutrients, see pages 9–13.

- Food allergies cause 20–30 percent of all eczema outbreaks. Common culprits include cow's milk, eggs, wheat, citrus fruits, chocolate, and shellfish. Try eliminating these foods from your child's diet one at a time to determine if a food allergy is behind the problem.
- Vitamin C helps reduce swelling and control eczema. Give your child 2 doses every day for up to 1 month.
- Vitamin E oil aids tissue healing and moisturizes the skin. Apply several drops of oil to the affected area once a day.
- Zinc promotes the healing of wounds, including eczema. Give your child 1 dose of zinc daily for several weeks.

Herbal

Use one or more of the remedies listed below.

- If the affected area is dry and scaly, apply calendula ointment. Follow directions for use provided on the product label.
- Evening primrose oil can be applied topically once a day to reduce inflammation and redness. It can also be taken internally; follow dosage directions on the package label.
- Oatmeal baths can help soothe itchy skin. Try a commercially prepared, powdered oatmeal treatment and follow package directions.

Homeopathy

Use one homeopathic treatment at a time, based on your child's specific symptoms. For dosage information, see the chart on page 25. Discontinue use if the symptoms disappear.

- *Graphites* 30x or 9c: Use if your child's skin is weepy and releasing a honey-colored pus behind the ears or on the palms of the hands. Give 1 dose 3 times a day for up to 5 days.
- *Mezereum (Daphne mezereum)* 6c: Use if your child has oozing crusty areas on the scalp. Give 1 dose 3 times daily for up to 5 days.
- *Rhus tox. (Rhus toxicodendron)* 6c: Use if your child's skin is blistered, especially around the wrists. Give 1 dose 3 times daily for up to 5 days.
- *Sulphur* 6c: Use if your child develops dry, itchy, red skin after bathing. Give 1 dose 4 times daily for up to 5 days.

Acupressure

Use one or more of the acupressure points listed below. For a diagram showing the specific pressure points, see pages 40–41.

- Heavenly Pillar (Bladder 10): This point is located a ½ inch below the base of the skull on the muscles a ½ inch outward from either side of the spine.
- Sea of Vitality (Bladder 23 and Bladder 47): To find this point, place your fingers in the lower back, between the second and third lumbar vertebrae, 2–4 child's finger widths away from the spine at waist level.
- Three Mile Point (Stomach 36): Apply steady pressure on the point 4 child's finger widths below the kneecap toward the outside of the shinbone.

An Ounce of Prevention

If your little one has sensitive skin, your goal is to avoid everything that irritates the skin or causes allergic reactions. Dress him in cotton clothes instead of wool, silk, or synthetics.

Keep the skin well moisturized by quick showers (or baths) and frequent applications of a moisturizer. If your child swims in a chlorinated pool, be sure he rinses thoroughly to remove all traces of the harsh chemicals.

When to Call for Help

The first time your child develops eczema, the condition should be diagnosed and treated by a doctor. Subsequent outbreaks can be treated at home, except when your child develops an open sore that shows signs of infection. Look for yellowish discharge or pus, swelling, and/or red streaks in the area of the site.

Fever

Fever is the body's way of fighting infection. When your child develops a fever, his body's immune system is responding to a bacterial or viral invasion. The body produces white blood cells and sends them out into the bloodstream to fight the invaders. The fever is not just a symptom of an illness, it is evidence that healing is occurring.

High fevers can lead to seizures or convulsions, especially in children with illnesses that cause a sudden, spiked fever. Febrile (fever) seizures occur in 3 to 5 percent of healthy children, usually in children between 6 months and 4 years of age. These seizures usually last 1–5 minutes; they should be brought to a doctor's attention immediately to rule out the possibility of a serious health problem.

Fever may be accompanied by a "chill." When your child has a fever, the complex system of temperature regulation in the body gets out of whack, and the perception of hot and cold gets skewed. Despite complaints that your child feels cold, don't wrap him in heavy blankets or you will further raise his body temperature. Instead, provide a light cotton sheet or thin blanket.

A temperature of 100–101 degrees F is considered mild, 102–104 moderate, and above 104 high. Temperatures above 106 are rare and require immediate medical care. A child in good health can tolerate a high temperature for several hours without the fever causing any ill effects, but the body begins to suffer cellular damage at extreme temperatures, usually those above 110 degrees.

Since high temperatures can affect health, contact your doctor if your child's fever continues climbing by the hour. In the meantime, take steps to control the fever and make your child more comfortable.

Traditional Treatments

Get a good reading. When it comes to body temperature, there's no such thing as normal. Don't fixate on 98.6 degrees F as the normal baseline; your child's healthy temperature may vary by fully one and a half degrees off the 98.6 mark. You also have to take timing into account: Your child's temperature varies throughout the day, bottoming out first thing in the morning and rising in response to clothing, excitement, anxiety, and, of course, activity. It generally peaks in late afternoon or early evening. To get the best reading, take your child's temperature a half hour after he quiets down or finishes a meal.

Know your thermometer. Different types of thermometers give slightly different readings. A rectal thermometer usually provides the most accurate readings for small children. (Lubricate the thermometer with petroleum jelly, then insert it about 1 inch into the rectum and hold it in place for 3 minutes. Talk to your child to comfort him during the process.) Once your child is 4 or 5, you can switch to an oral thermometer, which should be held under the tongue with the mouth shut for 4–5 minutes. Digital and electronic thermometers can provide faster readings, but they may be slightly lower (or higher) than readings from traditional mercury thermometers. To calibrate the readings, take your child's temperature using both the digital thermometer and a mercury thermometer and compare the results. In the future, you can use the faster, high-tech thermometer and adjust the reading as necessary.

Turn to acetaminophen. To lower the fever, give your child a dose of pediatric acetaminophen in liquid or tablet form; follow package directions for proper dosage. Never give your child under age 18 aspirin (including ''baby aspirin''), which can cause Reye's syndrome, a potentially fatal disease.

Try a soothing bath. You may be able to lower your child's temperature by giving him a lukewarm sponge bath. Fill a tub with tepid water (81–92 degrees F), have your child hop in, and sponge the water over his body. The water will evaporate on his skin, cooling the body gradually and naturally. Never try an alcohol bath because the alcohol can be absorbed through the skin, causing alcohol poisoning.

Keep those cool drinks coming. A feverish child loses body fluids because of elevated temperature and quickened breathing. Offer your child frequent drinks and clear fluids, such as soup and gelatin. Don't serve tea or colas, since these beverages encourage fluid loss.

Feed a fever? Offer your child a variety of nutritious meals, and leave it up to him to decide whether or not he feels like eating.

Sorry, no school. Keep your child home from school and other activities as long as he has an elevated fever. Once his temperature has returned to normal for 24 hours, it's safe to let him return to school and play.

Natural Remedies

All of the natural remedies listed below can be used to supplement conventional medical treatment.

Diet and Nutrition

Dosage varies according to age; see the chart on pages 14–15 to determine to correct dose for your child. For good food sources of particular nutrients, see pages 9–13.

- Vitamin C helps reduce inflammation and fight infection. Give your child 1 dose 3 times a day for 2 or 3 days.

Herbal
Use one or more of the remedies listed below. Dosage varies according to age; see the chart on page 25 to determine the correct dose for your child.

* Garlic can help relieve a fever associated with bacterial infection. Give your child 1 dose of odorless garlic twice a day for 3 days, or as directed on the product label.
* Ginger tea helps reduce fever associated with a cold or flu. Give your child 1 dose 3 times a day for 1 or 2 days. (If your child objects to the taste, mix the tea with apple juice.)
* Give your child a sponge bath, but add a hint of mint tea, lemon juice, or eucalyptus oil to the water.

Homeopathy
Use one homeopathic treatment at a time, based on your child's specific symptoms. For dosage information, see the chart on pages 31–37. Discontinue use if the symptoms disappear.

* *Aconite (Aconitum napellus)* 30x or 9c: Use if your child suddenly develops a fever, especially after being exposed to cold wind. Give 1 dose every 2 hours for up to 2 doses.
* *Belladonna (Atropa belladonna)* 15c or 30c: Use if your child develops a sudden fever, accompanied by chills. Give 1 dose every hour for up to 4 doses.
* *Gelsemium (Gelsemium sempervirens)* 30x or 9c: Use if your child develops a fever, in addition to feeling flushed and achy. Give 1 dose every 2 hours for up to 4 doses.
* *Phosphorus* 30x or 9c: Use if your child develops a fever accompanied by a cough. Give 1 dose every 2 hours for up to 4 doses.

Acupressure
Use one or more of the acupressure points listed below. For a diagram showing the specific pressure points, see pages 40–41.

* Active Pond (Triple Warmer 4): To find this point, place your fingers in the hollow in the center of the wrist case.

- Big Mound (Pericardium 7): Apply steady pressure on the point in the middle of the inside of the wrist crease.
- Crooked Pond (Large Intestine 11): This point is located on the forearm at the outside edge of the elbow crease.

An Ounce of Prevention

To avoid fever, your child must avoid infection. Keep your child away from sick friends and schoolmates, and teach good hand-washing practices to minimize the risk of illness.

When to Call for Help

Most fevers resolve themselves without medical intervention, but you should call your doctor if your feverish child has a convulsion or stiff neck, seems confused, is difficult to awaken from sleep, or experiences difficulty breathing. If the fever is accompanied by vomiting or diarrhea, or lasts longer than 72 hours, call your doctor to avoid the risk of dehydration.

Flu

Both the common cold and the flu are caused by viruses, and both involve a cough, fever, sore throat, and runny nose. But when your child has the flu, his symptoms—and complaints—will let you know you're dealing with more than the common cold. The flu involves the cold symptoms, plus chills, fatigue, red eyes, and sore muscles. Some kids also experience vomiting and diarrhea.

Unfortunately, there's nothing you can do but treat the symptoms and allow the virus to run its course. Antibiotics won't kill viruses, though they may be called in if your child develops an earache, or pneumonia, or some other secondary infection. Instead, you'll have to try to comfort your child and manage his symptoms one by one. (For more information on treating individual symptoms, see the sections on cough, page 125; fever, page 161; sore throat, page 249; and runny nose, page 246.)

Is It a Cold or the Flu?

Influenza and the common cold share certain characteristics, but there are ways to distinguish the two:

- *Fever*: Characteristic of the flu, but rare with a cold.
- *Headache*: Common with the flu, rare with a cold.
- *Achiness*: Severe with flu, slight with a cold.
- *Fatigue*: Severe and lingering with flu, minor with a cold.
- *Runny nose*: Minor with the flu, but characteristic of a cold.
- *Sore throat*: Possible with flu, common with a cold.
- *Cough*: Common with both flu and cold, but more severe with the flu.

Traditional Treatments

Turn down the heat. Give your child acetaminophen to bring down a high fever. Follow the package directions for proper dosage. Never give your child under age 18 aspirin (including "baby aspirin"), especially with the flu, since it can cause Reye's syndrome, a potentially fatal disorder.

Turn up the humidity. Moist air can help your child breathe. Run a humidifier or vaporizer in your child's bedroom at night. Be sure to clean the appliance regularly, following the manufacturer's directions.

Control the cough. During the day, let your child cough to bring up mucus and bacteria from the lungs. At night, if the cough interferes with your child getting a good night's sleep, consider using an over-the-counter cough suppressant.

Drink early, drink often. If you don't encourage your child to drink as much as possible, the high fever and possible vomiting can cause your child to become dehydrated. Offer water, clear soups, gelatin, diluted fruit juice, and flat ginger ale. During a bout of vomiting, offer fluids one teaspoon at a time. (Drinking too much fluid may cause the vomiting to continue.) If your child can't keep anything down, wait 15 or 20 minutes, and try again.

Natural Remedies

All of the natural remedies listed below can be used to supplement conventional medical treatment.

Diet and Nutrition
Dosage varies according to age; see the chart on pages 14–15 to determine the correct dose for your child. For good food sources of particular nutrients, see pages 9–13.

- Vitamin C with bioflavonoids helps fight viruses and reduce inflammation. Give your child 1 dose 3 times a day for 5 days.

Herbal
Use one or more of the remedies listed below. Dosage varies according to age; see the chart on page 25 to determine the correct dose for your child.

- Echinacea fights viruses, goldenseal fights bacteria, and both herbs boost the immune system. Give your child 1 dose of an echinacea and goldenseal formula 3 times a day for 4 or 5 days.
- Garlic helps fight infections. Give your child 1 dose of odorless garlic twice a day for 3 or 4 days.
- Ginger tea helps soothe an upset stomach. Give your child 1 dose of ginger tea as needed, for up to 3 days.

Homeopathy
Use one homeopathic treatment at a time, based on your child's specific symptoms. For dosage information, see the

chart on pages 31–37. Discontinue use if the symptoms disappear.

- *Arsenicum (Arsenicum album)* 30x or 9c: Use if your child feels weak, restless, and chilly. Give 1 dose 4 times a day for up to 3 days.
- *Eupatorium (Eupatorium perfoliatum)* 12x or 6c: Use if your child feels achy and tired. Give 1 dose 3–4 times a day for up to 3 days.
- *Mercurius (Mercurius solubilis hahnemanni)* 12x or 6c: Use if your child has a flu that lingers, accompanied by sore throat, and tender swollen glands. Give 1 dose 3 times a day for up to 3 days.

Acupressure

Use one or more of the acupressure points listed below. For a diagram showing the specific pressure points, see pages 40–41.

- Heavenly Rejuvenation (Triple Warmer 15): This point is located in the center of the shoulder blades, a ½ inch down the back from the top of the shoulders.
- Joining the Valley (Large Intestine 4): To find this point, place your fingers at the highest spot of the muscle on the back of the hand that protrudes when the thumb and index finger are close together. Once you locate the point, relax the fingers and apply pressure.
- Wind Mansion (Governing Vessel 16): Apply steady pressure on the point in the center of the back of the head, in the large hollow under the base of the skull.

An Ounce of Prevention

Flu shots (vaccinations against the current influenza strain) help prevent flu, but the shot itself can cause flu-like symptoms. Still, the federal Centers for Disease Control and Prevention in Atlanta recommends that kids with chronic illnesses, such as heart or lung disease, asthma, or diabetes, get flu shots every year since the flu can be fatal to people in poor health. Talk to your doctor about whether your child should be vaccinated.

When to Call for Help

Call the doctor if you suspect your child has the flu. The doctor should also be notified if your child experiences a fever-related convulsion, prolonged vomiting or diarrhea, difficulty in breathing, delirium, or infrequent urination. Sometimes the flu leads to serious complications, such as pneumonia or encephalitis, so contact your doctor if your child develops a cough that lasts more than 1 week or a stiff neck.

Food Poisoning

You can't see it, but if your child has it, you'll know it. A few hours after a meal, he will complain about a tummy-ache or cramping. Then the vomiting, diarrhea, and gas pains strike.

Food poisoning is a temporary problem with the stomach and intestinal tract that is caused by contaminated food. Most food poisoning is a result of staphylococci bacteria, the same nasty bugs that cause boils and impetigo. Other bacteria cause problems such as botulism or dysentery, but these infections tend to be less common.

In most cases, the contamination occurs during food preparation, and if the food is not properly refrigerated, the germs multiply and reach levels high enough to wreak havoc on your child's intestines. Starchy dishes, such as potato and pasta salads, provide a perfect petri dish for breeding bacteria. Since the germs can't be smelled or tasted, the unsuspecting diner has no idea that the food is acting as a poison to the body.

Most outbreaks of food poisoning show up 1 to 6 hours

after eating, though sometimes the symptoms don't appear for 24–48 hours. Usually, the condition lasts 12–24 hours, or until all the toxins have been eliminated from the body.

Traditional Treatments

Bottoms up. The vomiting and diarrhea associated with food poisoning cause the body to lose a tremendous amount of liquid. Encourage your child to sip water every few minutes to replenish those liquids. If the water stays down, switch to diluted fruit juices or sports drinks, which are more rapidly absorbed by the body because they contain sugar.

Skip meals. You child probably won't want to come anywhere near the dinner table for at least a day, which is perfectly okay. Introduce solid foods slowly, starting with bland foods, such as bananas, rice, applesauce, and toast. Give your child other foods when he feels ready.

Natural Remedies

All of the natural remedies listed below can be used to supplement conventional medical treatment.

Diet and Nutrition

- Lactobacillus acidophilus helps restore the beneficial bacteria to the intestinal tract. Give your child 1 dose 1 day after the outbreak, then 2 or 3 times a day for 5 days after that. Follow dosage information on the product label.

Herbal

Use one or more of the remedies listed below. Dosage varies according to age; see the chart on page 25 to determine the correct dose for your child.

- Garlic tablets help relieve the symptoms of food poisoning. Give your child 1 odorless garlic capsule twice a day for up to 2 days.

- Ginger tea soothes the stomach and helps clean out the digestive tract. Give your child 1 dose 3 times a day for up to 2 days.

Homeopathy

Use one homeopathic treatment at a time, based on your child's specific symptoms. For dosage information, see the chart on pages 31–37. Discontinue use if the symptoms disappear.

- *Baptisia (Baptisia tinctoria)* 6c: Use if your child's stools are dark, nearly liquid, and if he feels exhausted and wrung out. Give 1 dose every hour for up to 10 doses.
- *Colocynth (Citrullus colocynthis)* 6c: Use if your child experiences colicky pain that is relieved by gentle pressure on the abdomen. Give 1 dose every hour for up to 10 doses.
- *Phosphoric ac. (Phosphoricum acidum)* 6c: Use if your child's diarrhea is made worse when he moves, and if your child does not experience pain or vomiting. Give 1 dose every hour for up to 10 doses.

Acupressure

For a diagram showing the specific pressure point, see pages 40–41.

- Severe Mouth (Stomach 45): This point is located on the outside of the base of the nail of the second toe.

An Ounce of Prevention

You can't control the hygiene practices of food establishments away from home, but there are precautions you can take to minimize the risk of food poisoning in your own kitchen:

- The staphylococcus bacteria thrives on the skin and can easily contaminate food. Wash your hands with antibacterial soap before, during, and after preparing food. Wash again each time you handle raw meat, chicken, or eggs.
- Never leave food at room temperature for more than 2 hours, and throw out any food that sits out longer than that. You

want to keep food out of the bacteria-breeding temperature range—40 degrees–150 degrees F—as much as possible.

- After eating, immediately refrigerate leftovers. If the food is still hot, divide it into smaller portions or put in shallow containers, then pop them in the fridge. Don't wait for the food to cool before refrigerating it. Keep your refrigerator set to 40 degrees F, and the freezer set at 0 degrees F.
- Thaw meat and poultry in the refrigerator. Bacteria can grow on warm food surfaces, even though the center of the food may remain frozen.
- Don't serve or eat raw eggs, fish, fowl, or unpasteurized ("raw") milk. Skip making Caesar salad dressing with raw eggs, and pass up on eggnog made with unpasteurized eggs (the type of egg should be noted on a package of prepared eggnog). Sorry, no raw cookie dough, either.
- Cook food thoroughly: Cook red meat until it's no longer pink, poultry until the pink disappears and the juice runs clear, and fish until it flakes with a fork.
- Be wary of juice from raw meat. Take care that it does not drip on other foods in your shopping cart or refrigerator.
- Buy a separate cutting board to use with raw meat; rinse it with bleach after each use.
- If in doubt, throw it out. Never taste leftovers that have been in the back of the refrigerator for more than a few days, or foods that just don't "look right." Likewise, toss out dented cans, cracked jars, swollen containers, and other suspicious-looking food containers.

When to Call for Help

Food poisoning usually runs its course within a day or two, but the condition can be serious in young children. Contact your doctor if your child experiences severe vomiting or diarrhea for more than 12 hours for an infant, or 24 hours for a toddler or older child. Also contact your doctor if your child experiences bloody diarrhea, a fever above 100 degrees, difficulty swallowing or breathing, changes in vision, muscle weakness, paralysis, or prolonged abdominal pain.

Frostnip and Frostbite

Sledding, skiing, and building snowmen are some of the most wonderful activities a child can experience during winter, but rosy-cheeked and chilly can quickly become frostnipped or frostbitten, if you don't keep a watchful eye on your child's skin.

Frostnip and frostbite are caused by a lack of circulation in the hands, feet, ears, nose, and other extremities. When exposed to excessive cold, the blood vessels in these areas constrict and the blood thickens. With frostnip, the cold disrupts the pain messages sent by the nerves and the tissue feels numb. With frostbite, ice crystals form in the cell fluids, causing tissue damage. The skin may blister or peel several days after exposure.

Frostbitten skin appears white and waxy and feels hard to the touch. It can be quite painful when warmed. Frostbitten skin must be carefully and gradually thawed to minimize risk of permanent damage; the condition requires immediate medical attention. In rare cases of extreme frostbite, the frozen tissue dies and turns black and the damaged area must be amputated.

Traditional Treatments

- *Unwrap your child.* First, remove all cold, wet clothes so that you can assess the actual damage. The wet clothes draw body heat, so the sooner your child sheds his cold wraps, the sooner you can get to work on warming him up.
- *Easy does it.* Fill a bath with warm—not hot—water. (If the water is too warm, it can burn a child's sensitive skin, so try to limit the temperature to no more than 104–108 degrees F, or slightly warmer than body temperature.) Refresh the

water as necessary to keep it the appropriate temperature. It may take 15 or 20 minutes for the feeling to return to normal, so be patient.

- *Use kid gloves.* Handle the frostnipped tissue with great care. There are tiny ice crystals in the tissue, and rubbing the skin can slice and damage delicate tissue.
- *Use common sense.* Forget the old folk remedy of rubbing snow on frostbite; all it will do is cause the damaged tissue to freeze faster.

Natural Remedies

All of the natural remedies listed below can be used to supplement conventional medical treatment.

Herbal
Use one or more of the remedies listed below.

- Aloe cream helps heal blisters caused by frostbite. However, if frostbite is severe enough to cause the skin to blister, you should seek immediate medical attention.
- Cayenne pepper is an excellent vasodilator; it increases circulation to fingers, toes, and other extremities. Mix one teaspoon of cayenne pepper with 4 ounces of olive oil and rub it into the frostbitten skin.

Homeopathy
Use one homeopathic treatment at a time, based on your child's specific symptoms. For dosage information, see the chart on pages 31–37. Discontinue use if the symptoms disappear.

- *Apis (Apis mellifica)* 30c: Use if your child experiences severe burning pain when the skin is defrosted. Give 1 dose every 15 minutes for up to 6 doses. Apis lotion or ointment can also be applied topically.
- *Lachesis (Trigonocephalus lachesis)* 6c: Use if your child experiences purple or blue discoloration of the skin. Give 1 dose every 15 minutes for up to 6 doses.

An Ounce of Prevention

You can prevent frostnip and frostbite by dressing your child in multiple layers of cold-weather gear, including, of course, a hat, scarf, and mittens. Look for winter gear made of polypropylene and other synthetic fibers that "wick" moisture away from the skin, keeping skin dry and warm. Choose water-resistant mittens (which are warmer than gloves) and boots with removable liners that can be dried out between uses.

Layers trap warmth better than a single heavy coat because warm air is trapped between the many layers of clothing. The top layer should be made of a water-resistant fabric. Layers also allow your child to remove clothing as necessary to prevent becoming overheated and sweating, which can cause the skin to become damp and more easily chilled.

Also, call your children in from the cold to take a break and drink something hot every hour or so, depending on the temperature. Check for wet mittens and early signs of frostnip, such as stiff muscles and pale skin. Many kids won't notice that their fingers are getting numb, or they won't want to come in because they're having such a good time playing outside.

Take the windchill factor seriously. A blistering wind will cause the body to lose heat more quickly, even if the thermometer doesn't indicate extreme temperatures. For example, a 20-mile per hour wind on a 10 degree F day would result in a windchill factor of −25 degrees F—a temperature far too cold to permit outdoor play. Keep your kids indoors if the temperature or windchill falls more than 10 degrees below freezing.

When to Call for Help

Frostbite demands prompt medical attention to minimize risk of infection, or loss of fingers and toes. If you try the warm-water treatment and the affected area does not regain sensation and normal color within 15–20 minutes, call a doctor. Likewise, any frostbite that results in blisters or blue, swollen skin should be seen by a medical professional.

You also need to be on the alert for hypothermia, a potentially fatal condition where the body's temperature drops below 95 degrees F. If your child seems pale, confused, disoriented, or sleepy after being exposed to extreme cold, seek immediate medical attention.

Gas

It often happens at the most inopportune time: You place your infant or toddler before an attentive audience of friends and family, only for the sounds of admiration to be interrupted by a loud, unintentional intestinal outburst. Oops. While such episodes are to be expected, they can be quite embarrassing, as most parents know.

Flatulence (from the Latin word *flatus*, meaning blowing) is a normal part of the digestive process. Indeed, the average person releases nearly 1 quart of gas each day. Gas forms when undigested food passes from the small intestine into the large intestine and colon, where bacteria feast on the remains and give off noxious gases in the process. It can also be caused by swallowed air and food allergies. Babies tend to produce gas because they suck air when feeding and crying. Excessive and painful gassiness in babies is referred to as colic (see page 114).

Once it is trapped, gas has only two means of escaping—through belching or flatulating. Adults often find both options embarrassing, school-age kids often find both amusing, and babies and toddlers couldn't care less either way.

Traditional Treatments

- *No air, no wind.* One way to reduce gas is to reduce the amount of air your child swallows. Experiment with different bottles and nipple designs if your child drinks from a bottle. After feeding (or midway through a feeding), hold your baby upright and burp him thoroughly; air that doesn't makes its way up as a burp can cause a painful bubble if trapped down in the digestive tract. For the same reason, encourage your older children to relax and eat slowly to reduce the amount of air they take in.

- *How do you spell relief?* When it comes to beans, the answer may be B-E-A-N-O. This enzyme-based, anti-gas product really does help prevent the formation of gas when a few drops are placed on food before eating gas-producing foods. It's available at some supermarkets, pharmacies, and health food stores.
- *Skip the sorbitol.* Many sugar-free foods contain sorbitol, an artificial sweetener that contributes to the formation of gas. If your child has a problem with gas, teach him to just say no to sorbitol, which is found in diet foods.
- *Work it out.* Regular exercise helps keep the digestive system moving. After a meal, encourage your child to be active and help the body eliminate the gas before it builds up and causes unnecessary pain.

Natural Remedies

All of the natural remedies listed below can be used to supplement conventional medical treatment.

Diet and Nutrition
Use one or more of the remedies listed below.

- Monitor your child's diet, since some vegetables and complex carbohydrates are more likely than others to produce gas. Common culprits include beans, broccoli, brussels sprouts, cauliflower, cabbage, and onions. Don't eliminate these foods from your child's diet, but try cutting back on portion sizes if excessive gas is a problem, and see if you notice improvement.
- Milk and dairy products (except yogurt) can cause gas in children who are lactose intolerant (those whose bodies lack enough of the enzyme needed to digest milk sugars). If you

suspect a lactose problem, your doctor can confirm your diagnosis with a simple test. Supplemental enzymes are also available, and can eliminate the problem in many cases.

- Lactobacillus acidophilus helps with digestion and can ease gas pain by encouraging the growth of the "good" bacteria necessary for a healthy digestive system. Give your child 1 dose twice a day, following dosage information on the product label.

Herbal

Use one or more of the remedies listed below. Dosage varies according to age; see the chart on page 25 to determine the correct dose for your child.

- Garlic and ginger can minimize the impact of gas-producing foods such as beans. Use garlic and ginger regularly when preparing meals; it is also a nice complement to the flavor of many foods.
- Dill relaxes the muscles of the digestive tract. Add 1 teaspoon of dill seeds to 1 cup of boiling water, and let steep for 10 minutes. Give your child 1 or 2 tablespoons of this tea once a day.
- Fennel helps the body expel gas and aids in digestion. Add 1 teaspoon of fennel seeds to a cup of boiling water, and let steep for 10 minutes. Give your child 1 or 2 tablespoons of this tea once a day.
- Warm peppermint tea enhances digestion and acts as an antiflatulent. Give your child 1 teaspoon of peppermint tea, 4 to 5 times a day.

Acupressure

Use one or more of the acupressure points listed below. For a diagram showing the specific pressure points, see pages 40–41.

- Grandfather Grandson (Spleen 4): This point is located on the arch of the foot, 1 child's thumb width behind the ball of the foot.
- Sea of Energy (Conception Vessel 6): To find this point,

place your fingers 2 child's finger widths directly below the belly button.
- Three Mile Point (Stomach 36): Apply steady pressure on the point 4 child's finger widths below the kneecap, 1 finger width on the outside of the shinbone. If you are in the correct spot, a muscle should flex as the foot moves up and down.

An Ounce of Prevention

To some degree, you can control the frequency of gaseous outbursts by regulating your child's diet and eating habits. Encourage your child to eat slowly to minimize the amount of air he swallows. If flatulence is a frequent problem, look for signs of lactose intolerance (for more information, see page 202.)

When it comes to cooking dried beans, you can reduce their gas-producing potential by about 50 percent (without reducing their protein) by putting them through a series of soaks and rinses. First, rinse the beans. Then add them to boiling water for 3 minutes, turn off the heat, and let stand for 2 hours. Drain, then add more room-temperature water, enough to just cover the beans. After 2 hours, drain again, refill the water and let the beans soak overnight. Rinse one last time and the beans are ready to be cooked and used in the recipe of your choosing.

If you don't want to bother with this gas-reducing ritual, try using canned beans or switch to easier-to-digest varieties, such as split peas, limas, lentils, and Anasazi beans.

When to Call for Help

A bit of gas and occasional gas pains are nothing to worry about. However, a stubborn stomachache or abdominal pain (especially on the lower right-hand side) should be taken seriously, since it could be a sign of appendicitis. If in addition to gas pains your child has a fever, nausea, vomiting, or diarrhea, contact your pediatrician or other health care provider.

Headaches

When your head hurts, everything hurts. So when your child complains of a headache—as nearly 3 out of 4 children will at some point during childhood—try to be tolerant of their irritability and crankiness.

While there are a number of different causes of headaches, there are two main types: tension and migraine headaches. Tension headaches are characterized by a steady, dull pain starting at the front or back of the head, then spreading over the entire head. Migraine headaches, on the other hand, involve a throbbing, piercing, intense pain.

As the name implies, tension headaches usually stem from tension in the muscles of the face, neck, or scalp in response to stress or anxiety. The muscles squeeze the nerves and constrict the blood supply, causing pain and pressure. Relaxing the muscles eases the pain—if only it were that easy.

Migraine headaches begin to throb when the blood vessels in the head expand more than normal, often in response to food allergies, hormonal changes, stress, and other factors. Migraine pain can last for hours or days, and may be accompanied by nausea and vomiting. Migraines are a surprisingly common disorder, affecting an unfortunate 10 percent of the children who get headaches.

Traditional Treatments

Try a painkiller. A good first place to start in treating your child's headache is the medicine cabinet. Many headaches respond well to the painkillers acetaminophen and ibuprofen. Follow the package directions for dosage information. Never give your child under age 18 aspirin (including "baby aspirin''), because of the risk of developing Reye's syndrome, a potentially fatal brain and liver disorder.

Try a cool compress. Or a warm one. Wet a clean cloth and lay it across your child's forehead for 20–30 minutes. Let your child decide whether warm or cool water feels better. Lying down also may help your child relax. If bright light bothers your child's eyes, as it often does during a migraine, draw the shades and turn off the overhead lights.

Ahhh, massage. A gentle massage of the temples, scalp, neck, and shoulders may help relax the muscles and ease a tension headache. Of course, if your child wants to be left alone, honor his wishes or you'll make matters worse.

Try to identify the triggers. To find out what causes headaches—and therefore what can prevent them—carefully monitor your child's eating habits (for migraine) and behavior (for tension). Common food triggers for migraine include caffeine, chocolate, peanuts, aged cheese, processed meats, and food containing monosodium glutamate (MSG). Keep a food diary and look for links between what your child eats and what your child feels. Using the same approach, monitor your child's activities and look for emotional patterns between stress and headaches. Some children develop headaches before or after exams, or after having a fight with a friend. Talking to your child about stress and the underlying problem can help eliminate the tension headaches.

Take a break. Some kids spend hours transfixed by their computer screens, either playing video games or working on their homework. If your video lover develops tension headaches caused by muscle overuse, encourage him to take a 10-minute break every hour to roll his head, flex his shoulders, and stretch his legs with a short walk.

Natural Remedies

All of the natural remedies listed below can be used to supplement conventional medical treatment.

Diet and Nutrition

Use one or more of the remedies listed below. Dosage varies according to age; see the chart on pages 14–15 to determine to correct dose for your child. For good food sources of particular nutrients, see pages 9–13.

- Low blood sugar can cause dizziness and headaches. Give your child 3 nutritious meals a day, and healthy snacks between full meals, if necessary.
- Calcium and magnesium help relax the muscles and ease tension headaches. Give your child 1 dose of each twice a day for 2 or 3 days.

Herbal

Use one or more of the remedies listed below. Dosage varies according to age; see the chart on page 25 to determine the correct dose for your child.

- Chamomile tea helps calm the nervous system and relieve tension headache. Give your child 1 dose of tea.
- Ginger tea helps ease pain located in the forehead, caused by either tension or migraine headaches. Give your child 1 dose of tea.
- Skullcap relieves headaches caused by nervous tension. If your child is more than 6 years old, give 1 dose to relieve the pain.
- Tiger Balm liniment eases tension headaches. Rub the ointment into your child's temple area to relax the muscles, in response to the liniment and the rubbing action.

Homeopathy

Use one homeopathic treatment at a time, based on your child's specific symptoms. For dosage information, see the chart on pages 31–37. Discontinue use if the symptoms disappear.

- *Gelsemium (Gelsemium sempervirens)* 12x or 6c: Use if your child develops a tension headache. Give 1 dose every 20 minutes for 2 doses.
- *Iris (Iris versicolor)* 30x or 9c: Use if your child develops

a migraine headache, accompanied by impaired vision. Give 1 dose 4 times daily for up to 2 days.

- *Natrum mur. (Natrum muriaticum)* 30x or 9c: Use if your child develops a headache following a long period of focused mental work. Give 1 dose 4 times daily for up to 2 days.

Acupressure

Use one or more of the acupressure points listed below. For a diagram showing the specific pressure points, see pages 40–41.

- Drilling Bamboo (Bladder 2): This point is located in the indentations on either side of where the bridge of the nose meets the ridge of the eyebrows.
- Gates of Consciousness (Gallbladder 20): To find this point, place your fingers below the base of the skull, in the hollow just outside the two large, vertical neck muscles.
- Third Eye Point (Governing Vessel 24.5): Apply steady pressure on the point directly between the eyebrows, in the indentation where the bridge of the nose joins the forehead.
- Wind Mansion (Governing Vessel 16): This point is located in the center of the back of the head in a large hollow under the base of the skull.

An Ounce of Prevention

To avoid tension headaches, encourage your child to talk about emotional stresses (growing up can be hard on a child). If your child's headaches follow a meal that includes certain trigger foods, he probably has a food allergy, and you should avoid the foods that bring on headaches. If your child develops headaches when hungry, be sure to provide regular meals and healthy snacks throughout the day.

When to Call for Help

Most headaches amount to little more than an occasional inconvenience. In rare cases, however, headaches are warning signs of serious health problems, such as meningitis, encephalitis, or brain abnormalities. Call the doctor if the headache follows a head injury, immediately follows a sneeze or sudden cough, occurs each morning along with nausea, or if it is accompanied by fever, stiff neck, lethargy, or vomiting. Also call the doctor if the headaches become more severe over time or become a recurring problem (1 a week or more).

Heat Exhaustion and Heatstroke

Too much of a good thing can lead to trouble. Hot and humid summer heat, especially combined with vigorous play or exercise, can result in heat exhaustion or heatstroke.

The human body is designed to defend itself against adversity, including excessive heat. When exposed to high temperatures and humidity, the body tries to cool itself by sending blood to the skin's surface, causing the common flush associated with being overheated. For the same reason, the body also releases sweat, which cools the body as it evaporates on the skin.

The system works well, except when the body is heated for too long. When too much blood has been sent away from the body's inner core, dizziness, confusion, fainting or even coma can result. Too much sweat can cause dehydration, which causes the body to stop producing sweat to conserve fluids, leaving the body further unable to cool itself.

The first symptoms of heat exhaustion are dizziness and nausea, followed by a racing heartbeat, muscle cramps, and rapid, shallow breathing. At this early stage, the core body temperature has risen only slightly, and the condition is not usually serious if your child is cooled down promptly.

If the overheating is not addressed, however, heat exhaustion can turn into heatstroke (also known as sunstroke). At this point, the body becomes dehydrated and stops sweating. The core body temperature continues to rise, often to 106 degrees F or higher, and the person collapses and falls into a coma. Heatstroke is a medical emergency with a 10–20 percent fatality rate, even among healthy people who receive medical care.

Traditional Treatments

- *If you can't stand the heat . . .* Get your child out of the sun. On hot days, ask your child to play in the shade, in a pool, or even indoors. If your child shows signs of overheating—dizziness, nausea, muscle cramps, rapid heartbeat, and shallow breathing—get him out of the direct sun to begin cooling him down. Move into an air-conditioned room or one with a fan, if possible.
- *Drink up.* At the first sign of overheating, give your child plenty of fluids. The fluids can help prevent dehydration and any further complications.
- *Time for a cool bath.* Submerge your child in cool—not cold water—to help lower his temperature. Elevate his feet by about 12 inches, and rub his legs and feet to aid circulation. If you can't put your child in a tub, apply cold water compresses to the back of the neck, inside of the wrists, and forehead to help lower the body temperature. Don't try an alcohol bath; the alcohol creates a cooling sensation, but it is absorbed through the skin and can be toxic.

Natural Remedies

All of the natural remedies listed below can be used to supplement conventional medical treatment.

Herbal

- As stated above, cool compresses help lower the body's temperature. Some people find the treatments even more effective if 10–12 drops of eucalyptus, peppermint, or lavender oil is added to each quart of cool water. The scents don't lower the temperature any faster, but they can be soothing and refreshing.

Homeopathy

Use one homeopathic treatment at a time, based on your child's specific symptoms. For dosage information, see the chart on pages 31–37. Discontinue use if the symptoms disappear.

- *Cuprum (Cuprum metallicum)* 6c: Use for muscle cramps. Give 1 dose every 5 minutes for up to 10 doses.
- *Belladonna (Atropha belladonna)* 30c: Use if the skin is flushed, hot, and dry, or if the pulse is strong and rapid. Give 1 dose every 5 minutes for up to 10 doses.

Acupressure

For a diagram showing the specific pressure point, see pages 40–41.

- One Hundred Meeting Point (Governing Vessel 20): To find this point, place your left fingers behind your child's left ear, and your right fingers behind your child's right ear. Move your fingertips to the top of his head, then feel for the hollow toward the back of the top center of your child's head.

An Ounce of Prevention

Heat exhaustion and heatstroke can be prevented. Start by exercising common sense: Get your child out of the midday sun. Make sure he comes inside for a cooldown several times during the afternoon. Though it should go without saying, *never* leave your child in a locked car, even for just a minute. Cars heat up to dangerous levels very quickly.

Be sure that your child drinks plenty of fluids. Encourage

your child to drink before, during, and after exercise. Every hour, an eight-year-old should drink an 8-ounce glass of water, juice, or a diluted electrolyte sports drink. (Older kids should drink up to 4 ounces more; younger kids, 4 ounces less.) Waiting for your child to be thirsty is not a good enough signal; his body will start to dehydrate long before it will register thirst.

When to Call for Help

Heat exhaustion demands immediate treatment to prevent it from escalating into heatstroke. Consider it an immediate medical emergency and seek emergency room treatment if your child is overheated and develops any of the following warning signs:

- weakness or lethargy
- headache
- fever of 104 degrees or more
- coma or convulsions
- disorientation or confusion

Immediately get your child out of the sun and begin to cool him off, using the techniques described above.

Hiccups

Hiccups remain one of the great mysteries of the human body: No one knows why we do it or how to make it stop. Some of the greatest minds in medicine have pondered the issue; the best advice Hippocrates could come up with was that sneezing could put an end to the annoying little spasms.

A hiccup is nothing more than an involuntary contraction of the diaphragm, which causes the vocal cords to shut and make the "hic" sound. Hiccups have been blamed on eating too fast, swallowing air, indigestion, and fatigue, but the exact physiological trigger is unknown.

People hiccup throughout their lives and even before they are born. Pregnant women often report that their babies hiccup several times a day in utero, and they continue in infancy. Hiccups are almost always harmless, and children often find them quite amusing.

Traditional Treatments

Alas, there is no surefire cure for hiccups. Most remedies work—some of the time—by either stimulating the nerve impulses in the throat or by increasing carbon dioxide levels in the blood. Hiccups usually vanish on their own in a few minutes, but if your child finds them disturbing try one or more of the remedies listed below:

For Babies

- Burp the baby to get rid of trapped air, especially if the hiccups appear after eating.
- Encourage your baby to sip some sugar water.

For Older Kids

- Have your child swallow a teaspoon of dry sugar. (A lot of kids like giving this remedy a try.)
- Ask your child to take a deep breath and hold it as long as possible.
- Encourage your child to breathe into a paper bag. (Don't try this with a child under age 3, who should not be taught to put bags over their heads).
- Have your child gargle with sugar water for 2 minutes.
- Ask your child to lean over and sip cold water from the opposite rim of a glass.
- Have your child pull his tongue and hold it for 1 minute.

- Startle your child, in attempt to "scare" the hiccups out of him.
- Squirt lemon juice down the back of your child's throat.

Natural Remedies

All of the natural remedies listed below can be used to supplement conventional medical treatment.

Homeopathy

For dosage information, see the chart on pages 31–37. Discontinue use if the symptoms disappear.

- *Nux (Strychnos nux vomica)* 6c: Use for hiccups accompanied by belching, especially after eating a large meal. Give 1 dose every 15 minutes for up to 1 hour.

Acupressure

Use one or more of the acupressure points listed below. For a diagram showing the specific pressure points, see pages 40–41.

- Abdominal Sorrow (Spleen 16): This point is located on the lower edge of the rib cage a ½ inch in from the nipple line.
- Center of Power (Conception Vessel 12): Apply steady pressure on the point along the center line of the body, 3 child's finger widths below the base of the breastbone.
- Letting Go (Lung 1): To find this point, place your fingers on the outer part of the chest, 2 inches above the crease of the armpit and 1 inch inward. When your child pulls his arm close to his body, you should feel a muscle bulge.
- Wind Screen (Triple Warmer 17): This point is located in the indentation behind the earlobe.

An Ounce of Prevention

There's no surefire way to prevent hiccups, since no one knows exactly why we hiccup in the first place. However, you may be able to avoid a few episodes of hiccuping by insisting that your children eat slowly to avoid swallowing excessive air during mealtime.

When to Call for Help

In the vast majority of cases, hiccups disappear within 5 or 10 minutes, leaving your child no worse for wear. That's not to say they won't ever last longer: Cases have been reported of hiccups lasting hours, weeks, and in very few cases, years. If your little one hiccups for more than a day, call your doctor. Persistent hiccups could be a symptom of a more serious health problem, such as a gastrointestinal blockage.

Hives

It could be almost anything: an allergy to a food or medication your child has taken, a bug bite, a reaction to a plant he brushed past when walking to school, or even a psychological response to personal stress or tension. Hives—patches of itchy, raised red bumps—can appear out of nowhere, and can disappear just as swiftly, though they sometimes linger for weeks at a time.

Hives form when the body releases histamine, a chemical in the body that causes the blood vessels to release clear fluid under the skin, forming blister-like welts. This histamine reaction is a natural response to irritation. In most cases, hives can be handled at home without complications.

Traditional Treatments

- *Stop the itching.* Try an over-the-counter oral antihistamine to ease the itch. Follow the package instructions. If your child becomes agitated or nervous in reaction to the drug, ask your doctor about substitute drugs.

- *Take a bath.* To ease your child's itchy hives, soak him in a warm bath spiked with a ½ cup of baking soda or an oatmeal bath product, such as Aveeno. If 1 bath doesn't do the trick, bathe him again later in the day.
- *Too cool to scratch.* The cool relief of an ice pack or cold compress can ease the urge to itch. Soak a clean washcloth in cool water and apply it to the hives for 10–15 minutes. Try this cool compress trick up to once an hour.

Natural Remedies

All of the natural remedies listed below can be used to supplement conventional medical treatment.

Herbal
Use one or more of the remedies listed below.

- Parsley inhibits the body's release of histamines, which cause hives and other allergic symptoms. Add additional parsley to food while cooking, or encourage your child to eat a few springs of fresh parsley with his meal.
- A paste of crushed chickweed leaves can ease itchy skin. Mix the powder with enough water to form a paste, and apply it directly to the hives. Reapply after it crumbles and starts falling off.

Homeopathy
Use one homeopathic treatment at a time, based on your child's specific symptoms. For dosage information, see the chart on pages 31–37. Discontinue use if the symptoms disappear.

- *Apis (Apis mellifica)* 30c: Use if your child develops hives or swollen lips and eyelids. Give 1 dose every hour for up to 5 doses.
- *Rhus tox. (Rhus toxicodendron)* 6c: Use for burning and itchy hives with blisters. Give 1 dose every hour for up to 5 doses.

- *Urtica (Urtica wrens)* 6c: Use if your child develops hives probably caused by a plant. Give 1 dose every hour for up to 5 doses.

Acupressure

Use one or more of the acupressure points listed below. For a diagram showing the specific pressure points, see pages 40–41.

- Heavenly Appearance (Small Intestine 17): This point is located in the indentation directly below the earlobe and behind the jawbone.
- Three Mile Point (Stomach 36): To find this point, place your fingers 4 child's finger widths below the kneecap toward the outside of the shinbone.
- Wind Screen (Triple Warmer 17): Apply steady pressure on the point in the indentation directly behind the earlobe.

An Ounce of Prevention

To prevent hives, you must determine what causes them in the first place. Unfortunately, that's much easier said than done. Doctors or allergists can identify the offending allergen that causes the outbreak in approximately 1 out of 4 cases. Still, if your child suffers chronic hives, you should consider seeking a physician's help in tracking down the cause. Also, keep track of your child's diet and exposure to animals and medications. Make a list of laundry detergents, household cleaners, and other possible chemicals to which your child is exposed. The more information you can provide to the doctor or allergist, the better your chances of identifying the culprit and ridding your child of hives.

When to Call for Help

While most episodes involving hives present no significant health risk, some allergic reactions can be potentially life-threatening. If in addition to the hives, your child's hands, feet, face and lips swell, or if your child complains that he can't swallow, contact your doctor and go to the emergency room immediately. Such a severe reaction can cause the tongue and throat to swell, which can block the airway. Your child will need a shot of adrenaline to reduce the swelling.

Hoarseness and Laryngitis

Most children have no trouble being heard—unless they come down with either a case of hoarseness or of laryngitis. Suddenly, whispers replace the wails and whines, at least for a few days.

With laryngitis, the upper part of the windpipe holding the vocal cords (the larynx) becomes swollen and tender. Due to the swelling, when your child tries to speak, the air being pushed out of his lungs no longer vibrates the same way as it normally does as it crosses the larynx. The result: Your child's distinctive voice is altered (hoarseness) or quieted entirely (laryngitis).

The swelling can be caused by a viral or bacterial infection, an allergic reaction, or simple overuse from a hard day of yelling on the soccer field. You can help soothe and restore your child's weary voice by following a few simple steps.

Traditional Treatments

Silence is healing. The less strain your child puts on his vocal cords, the faster the swelling will go down and his voice will return to normal. Communicate through written messages, pictures, or charades—anything but the spoken word.

Speak up. Contrary to popular belief, whispering strains the vocal cords as much as shouting. When your child must speak, encourage him to speak in an everyday tone of voice.

Keep it moist. Encourage your child to sip lukewarm water throughout the day, drink warm decaffeinated tea, and spoon down chicken soup, all of which can soothe an irritated throat. Throat lozenges or hard candies stimulate saliva flow, which aids in relieving a dry or irritated throat.

Take advantage of "mist" opportunities. Inhaling warm steam for 5 or 10 minutes at a time will soothe the throat and help clear away mucus. Use a vaporizer or humidifier in your child's bedroom at night, and sit with your child in a steamy bathroom 3 or 4 times a day. (If you use a humidifier or vaporizer, clean it often, following the manufacturer's instructions for doing so.)

Pretend you're underwater. Kids above age 5 or 6 should be able to gargle, and most will find the experience a great deal of fun. Gargling with saltwater (1 teaspoon of salt in an 8-ounce glass of warm water) can soothe the vocal cords. If your child is new to gargling, practice with plain water before attempting the salty version.

Natural Remedies

All of the natural remedies listed below can be used to supplement conventional medical treatment.

Herbal
Use one or more of the remedies listed below. Dosage varies according to age; see the chart on page 25 to determine the correct dose for your child.

- Garlic helps fight both viral and bacterial infections. Give your child 2 or 3 odorless garlic capsules a day for 2 or 3 days.
- To soothe the throat, have your child gargle with strong tea made with slippery elm. (Only try this if your child has practice gargling and spitting without swallowing. You do not want your child to ingest the tea.)
- Echinacea tea helps fight both viral and bacterial infections and boosts the immune system. Bring 2 teaspoons of echinacea root and 1 cup of water to a boil, then simmer 15 minutes. Give your child 1 dose of tea 3 times daily for 2 or 3 days. If you use a commercial preparation, follow the

package directions. WARNING: *Do not give echinacea to children under age two.*

Homeopathy

Use one homeopathic treatment at a time, based on your child's specific symptoms. For dosage information, see the chart on pages 31–37. Discontinue use if the symptoms disappear.

- *Arnica (Arnica montana)* 30c: Use if your child experiences voice loss due to straining or overuse. Give 1 dose 4 times daily for up to 7 days.
- *Phosphorus* 6c: Use if your child's throat feels dry and sore, and he has a painful cough that becomes worse near bedtime. Give 1 dose 4 times daily for up to 7 days.
- *Spongia (Spongia tosta)* 6c: Use if your child develops a dry, barking cough, as well as loss of his voice. Give 1 dose 4 times daily for up to 7 days.

Acupressure

Use one or more of the acupressure points listed below. For a diagram showing the specific pressure points, see pages 40–41.

- Crooked Pond (Large Intestine 11): This point is located on the forearm at the outer edge of the elbow crease.
- Elegant Mansion (Kidney 27): To find this point, place your fingers in the hollow below the collarbone next to the breastbone.

An Ounce of Prevention

Shhhhh. Strictly enforce the rule against yelling in the house and encourage your child to speak softly and avoid straining his voice when away from home. If the problem is exacerbated by dry winter air, run a humidifier in your child's room and throughout the house to keep the air moist, especially at night. Cigarette smoke can irritate the larynx, so avoid smoking around your child.

When to Call for Help

Voice changes in children under age 4 should be taken seriously and demand immediate medical attention, since their air passages are narrow and can easily become blocked or swollen shut. With older children, hoarseness rarely interferes with breathing, so there is no immediate need to contact a physician. Contact your doctor if your child experiences labored breathing, has a barking cough (see the section on croup on page 131), or difficulty swallowing (with lots of drool pooling in his mouth). In addition, give the doctor a call if your child has run-of-the-mill hoarseness that fails to clear up within 1 week.

Impetigo

You thought your worries were over when your child stopped complaining about that skinned knee or scratch from the dog. If impetigo sets in, your troubles are just beginning.

Impetigo is a highly contagious bacterial skin infection that can be caused by either the streptococcus or staphylococcus bacteria. When the bacteria enter your child's body through a break in the skin, small blisters appear, then scab over and form an itchy, yellow-brown crust that looks a bit like brown sugar.

In most cases, impetigo shows up around the nose and mouth, but it can appear on (or spread to) any part of the body. Touching the blisters, then touching another part of the body (or another person) can spread the infection. So can sharing washcloths or other linens used by the infected child.

Small outbreaks can be treated with an antibiotic ointment, but more severe outbreaks may require oral antibiotics. Your child remains contagious for the first 3 days of antibiotic treatment, so he should avoid unnecessary contact with other children before and during that time. After treatment, the condition should disappear within a week or two.

Traditional Treatments

- *Cleanliness is next to healthiness.* You can't keep the infected area too clean. Wash it with antibacterial soap at least 3 times a day.
- *Let it breathe.* Fresh air can help fight the bacteria. Covering the area with a bandage creates a moist, dark environment where the bacteria will thrive. One exception to this rule: If your child is going to play outside, cover the area during play, then remove the bandage when your child is back indoors.
- *Keep your hands to yourself.* Teach your child to avoid scratching whenever possible, and to wash his hands with soap and water regularly. Impetigo is often spread by bacteria trapped under the fingernails. Keep your child's nails short to help deter scratching.
- *Soak away the itch.* Cool baths or compresses can help ease the itch. In general, warm temperatures and heat increase itching, so try to keep your child from getting overheated, whenever possible.
- *Try an antihistamine.* When your child just can't stand the itching anymore, give him a dose of antihistamine, which will reduce itching and inflammation. (Check package directions for dosage information.)

Natural Remedies

All of the natural remedies listed below can be used to supplement conventional medical treatment.

Diet and Nutrition

Use one or more of the remedies listed below. Dosage varies according to age; see the chart on pages 14–15 to determine the correct dose for your child. For good food sources of particular nutrients, see pages 9–13.

- Vitamin C helps heal the skin and enhance the immune system. Give your child 1 dose 3 times a day for 7–10 days.
- Zinc helps boost the immune system and heal wounds. Give your child 1 dose once or twice a day for 7–10 days.

Herbal
Use one or more of the remedies listed below.

- Goldenseal powder helps fight infection and heal the rash common to impetigo. Mix the powder with a bit of warm water to form a paste and apply directly to the rash once or twice a day for 3 or 4 days.
- Apply calendula ointment to the rash twice a day.
- Tea tree oil has strong antibacterial and antifungal properties. Dilute 8–10 drops of tea tree oil in 1 quart of warm water and apply the mixture to the infected area twice a day.

Homeopathy
Use one homeopathic treatment at a time, based on your child's specific symptoms. For dosage information, see the chart on pages 31–37. Discontinue use if the symptoms disappear.

- *Antimonium (Antimonium crudum)* 6c: Use if your child has blisters around the nose and mouth. Give 1 dose every hour for up to 8 doses.
- *Arsenicum (Arsenicum album)* 30x or 9c: Use if your child has blisters and fatigue. Give 1 dose every hour for up to 6 hours.
- *Mezereum (Daphne mezereum)* 12x or 6c: Use if your child's scalp is affected with blisters that are encrusted and oozing. Give 1 dose every hour for up to 8 doses.

An Ounce of Prevention

You can usually prevent impetigo by treating a wound at the first sign of infection, so that the bacteria doesn't have a chance to enter the body. To avoid outbreaks around the face and nose when your child has a cold, lubricate the area with petroleum jelly to keep the skin moist and healthy.

When to Call for Help

If your child is less than a year old, call your doctor if you suspect he has impetigo. With older children, impetigo usually responds to home treatment, though severe cases demand a doctor's attention. Contact your pediatrician if there is a blister more than 1 inch across, or if your child develops a fever. Antibiotics may be needed to clear the infection.

In rare cases, infections of strep bacteria can cause a serious kidney disease. Call your doctor immediately if your child's urine becomes red or dark brown. Antibiotics will be needed to fight the infection.

Insect Bites and Stings

Kids can be as pesky to bugs as bugs are to grown-ups. And when kids bug the bugs, the bugs often bite back. Insects bite and sting to defend themselves. Most of the time these attacks amount to little more than a bothersome bump or itch, but other times they can be very serious.

For most children, a common insect bite or sting is little more than a short-term annoyance. But those who experience systemic allergic reactions may respond with asthma attacks (difficulty breathing and wheezing), hives and rashes, and fainting. If your child experiences a systemic reaction, you should assume that a comparable—or more severe—reaction will occur the next time he is bitten or stung.

In most cases, the insect venom consists of a complex combination of proteins and enzymes, which can affect a number of different organs. An individual's reaction to a bite or sting depends on a number of factors, including: the size of the child, the number and location of the stings or bites, and the body chemistry and allergic history of the person who was attacked. Obviously, the best way to avoid trouble is to leave the insects alone. But if your child does have a run-in with an angry insect, the following remedies can help.

Traditional Treatments

Get the stinger out. Wasps, hornets, and yellow jackets can sting repeatedly, without leaving their stingers behind. But if a honeybee or bumblebee (the ones with the fuzzy bodies) sting your child, the barbed stinger—along with its venom sac—will be left behind. Yanking on the stinger can cause more venom to pump into your child, so take a piece of cardboard, a credit card, or a long fingernail and scrape the stinger out.

Clean it up. Thoroughly wash any insect bite or sting with soap and water, and wash the area 3 or 4 times a day until it heals. Apply an antibiotic ointment to the wound after it is cleaned. There is no need to cover the area with a bandage, since the puncture wound is so small.

Ice it down. To ease the itch and deaden the pain, apply ice or an ice pack wrapped in a clean towel for 20–30 minutes. If your child complains that the ice is too cold, rinse a clean washcloth in cold water and use it as a compress instead.

Haven't got time for the pain. Acetaminophen can help relieve pain. Follow the package directions for dosage information. And never give aspirin (including "baby aspirin") to your child under age 18 because it can cause Reye's syndrome, a potentially fatal brain and liver disorder.

Get the itch out. You can try several treatments to ease the itch and relieve the pain. Dab a bit of household ammonia on the bite or sting. Or mix baking soda or meat tenderizer with just enough water to form a paste. (Use either baking soda *or* meat tenderizer, not both.) Apply the paste to the bite or sting and leave it for 15–20 minutes, then rinse. Antihistamines can also be used to relieve the itching. Follow the package directions for dosage information.

Natural Remedies

All of the natural remedies listed below can be used to supplement conventional medical treatment.

Diet and Nutrition

• Vitamin E helps bites and stings heal faster. Apply the oil directly to the site.

Herbal

Use one or more of the remedies listed below.

• Comfrey helps ease the itching and pain of insect bites, especially spider bites. Mix 3 tablespoons of powdered comfrey with 3 ounces of hot water. Apply the paste directly to the bite and cover the area with a bandage or sterile gauze pad. Leave paste on overnight. *Do not use internally.*
• Tea tree oil kills germs and promotes healing. Apply a few drops of oil directly to the bite or sting after washing thoroughly.

Homeopathy

Use one homeopathic treatment at a time, based on your child's specific symptoms. For dosage information, see the chart on pages 31–37. Discontinue use if the symptoms disappear.

• *Arnica (Arnica montana)* 30c: Use if your child develops swelling, bruising, and pain. Give 1 dose every 5 minutes for up to 10 doses.
• *Cantharis (Cantharis lytta vesicatoria)* 30c: Use after a bee sting. Give 1 dose every 15 minutes for up to 6 doses.
• *Carbolic ac. (Carbolic acidum)* 6c: Use if your child feels weak or collapses after a bee sting while also seeking emergency treatment. Give 1 dose every 15 minutes for up to 6 doses.
• *Crotalus (Crotalus horridus)* 6c: Use if your child experiences rapid onset of swelling and subcutaneous bleeding, with the skin around the bite becoming discolored. Give 1 dose every 5 minutes for up to 10 doses.

Acupressure
For a diagram showing the specific pressure point, see pages 40–41.

- Crooked Pond (Large Intestine 11): This point is located on the forearm at the outer edge of the elbow crease.

An Ounce of Prevention

Bug repellents, especially those containing DEET (diethyltoluamide), really work against mosquitoes, flies, bees, wasps, and other airborne irritants. Avon's Skin-So-Soft bath oil also discourages bugs, and it's safe to use on small children.

Teach your child not to swat at bees and wasps, which usually only sting when provoked. Instead, tell your child to freeze until the insect flies away. To discourage bees from approaching your child in the first place, avoid bright colored fabrics (especially floral prints), which attract bees. Also avoid perfumes and scented soaps, which can attract bees in search of sweet-smelling flowers.

When to Call the Doctor

If your child is allergic to bees, a sting should be considered a medical emergency. Seek immediate medical help if after a bee sting your child experiences difficulty breathing, tightness of the throat or chest, dizziness or fainting, nausea or vomiting, or swelling over a large part of his body. Even if your child is not allergic to bee stings, contact a doctor if your child is stung in the mouth or nose because the swelling can block the airways.

Children with bee allergies should be given a prescription emergency kit, containing antihistamines and injectable adrenaline. You should keep this potentially life-saving kit with your child when he is outdoors.

Some spider bites also demand immediate medical attention. Bites from the black widow and the brown recluse can be fatal. If you're not sure what kind of spider bit your child, seek immediate medical help. In addition, call the doctor after a spider bite if your child experiences muscle spasms, stiffness, or abdominal pain (symptoms of black widow bite) or a strange red, white, and blue bull's-eye rash around the bite, with blue or purple near the bite (symptoms of a brown recluse bite). Poisonous spider bites can also cause headache, fever, lethargy, and joint pain.

Lactose Intolerance

It happens every time: Your child drinks a glass of milk, munches on a slice of cheese pizza, or downs a bowl of Rocky Road ice cream—and then the problems begin. Within an hour or so, your child complains of gas and bloating, followed by a painful bout of diarrhea. The symptoms pass within a couple of hours, only to return the next time your child eats dairy products. As you may have determined by now, you child has lactose intolerance.

Lactose intolerance stems from a deficiency in lactase, an enzyme in the small intestine needed to absorb and digest lactose, the sugar in dairy products. Without a sufficient supply of lactase, when your child drinks milk, eats ice cream, or consumes other dairy products (except yogurt with live cultures), the lactose ferments and causes a multitude of unpleasant side effects throughout the digestive system. The condition is far from rare; in fact, about 70 percent of the world's population can't consume dairy products without paying for it a little bit later.

A child with lactose intolerance will grow into an adult with the same condition. However, some children develop a temporary problem handling dairy products when they suffer from an illness that causes their intestinal bacteria to get out of whack. If your child experiences signs of lactose intolerance during or after a round with a flu bug, don't despair. Your child may not be lactose intolerant but merely have a weak digestive system after struggling to fight off a bug. Actual lactose intolerance has no connection to intestinal illness; it is a problem within the digestive system itself. However, there are a number of steps you can take to help your child manage the condition.

Traditional Treatments

Find out what you're up against. If you suspect lactose intolerance (or another food allergy), keep a detailed log of the food your child eats and how he feels for 2 or 3 hours after eating. Your goal is to determine which foods trigger the digestive problems.

Mix it up. Experiment with your child's diet, trying to mix dairy foods with nondairy foods. For example, rather than drinking a glass of milk alone, offer your child a small glass of milk and a bagel with peanut butter. The nondairy foods dilute the milk sugar and arrive at the intestines over a longer period, reducing the risk of overpowering the enzymes that may be left in your child's intestine.

Get by with a little help from your druggist. You can buy over-the-counter lactase supplements that assist the body's own enzymes in breaking down milk sugars. These products, available in most drugstores, can be mixed with regular milk and/or taken alone.

Natural Remedies

All of the natural remedies listed below can be used to supplement conventional medical treatment.

Diet and Nutrition
Use one or more of the remedies listed below. Dosage varies according to age; see the chart on pages 14–15 to determine to correct dose for your child. For good food sources of particular nutrients, see pages 9–13.

- Unlike other dairy products, yogurt is safe for kids with lactose intolerance because the lactose is digested by the bacterial cultures in the yogurt before it reaches your stomach. (Just make sure the yogurt contains live cultures.)
- Children who cannot consume dairy products may need a calcium supplement to ensure an adequate intake of this important nutrient, which is crucial for bone development.

An Ounce of Prevention

Lactose intolerance cannot be prevented or permanently treated; instead, your child must learn to live with it. Teach your child to read food labels and look for lactose-containing ingredients, including milk, milk solids, cheese, whey, or lactose. When eating out, don't be shy about asking the waiter or chef whether a dish contains dairy products. Many digestive disasters can be avoided by painstakingly scrutinizing what goes into your child's mouth.

When to Call for Help

If you suspect lactose intolerance, talk the problem over with your doctor. Your pediatrician may want to perform some tests to determine just how sensitive your child's digestive system is, in addition to working with you to develop a diet that will provide plenty of calcium from nondairy food sources.

Lice

Don't take it personally; it happens in the best of families. Head lice afflict about 10 million people every year, and nearly 7 million cases involve children under the age of 12. Sooner or later, chances are good that one of them will be one of yours.

Look for lice if your child complains of an itchy scalp or if you spot him scratching incessantly. Sit your child down and separate the hair, looking closely for tiny, gray bumps (the lice) or grayish-white eggs that have become attached to the hair shaft near the scalp (the nits).

A lice infestation (known as *pediculosis* in medical parlance) has nothing to do with personal hygiene. In fact, lice prefer clean hair over the greasy stuff. Lice can spread through sharing brushes and combs, borrowing a hat or scarf, even just playing side by side.

It's easier to get lice than to get rid of them, but delousing your child shouldn't be too great a problem, provided you tend it right away. A sexually mature louse lays about 5 eggs a day, and those eggs hatch within 2 weeks, so if you wait too long to treat the problem, you will be facing a much more formidable enemy.

Traditional Treatments

- *Of lice and men.* Getting rid of lice requires some persistence—and some pesticides. Over-the-counter lice products come as shampoos, liquids, and gels. Follow the package instructions down to the letter; these treatments contain serious chemicals that should be treated with respect.
- *You're such a nit-picker.* And the pickier you are, the better off your child will be. The lice treatment will kill the active

lice, but not the nits. Getting rid of the nits reduces the chances of reinfestation, so go over your child's hair with a fine-toothed comb, literally. (Many lice treatments include a comb in the package.)

- *It's a family affair.* Where there is one louse, there will soon be many lice. You can save yourself the trouble of long cycles of lice treatment and reinfestation by treating everyone for lice at the same time.

- *Not a louse in the house.* Lice don't restrict their activity to your child's head, unfortunately. In addition to banishing them from the scalp, you must wash (hot water) and dry (high heat) everything you can that might have come in contact with your child's scalp. Include hats, coats, scarves, sheets, pillowcases, towels—if in doubt, wash it out. Thoroughly wash sofas, mattresses, rugs, and carpets. Wash combs, brushes, and hair barrettes in soapy water, then soak them in scalding water for 15 minutes.

- *Don't forget the toys.* Alas, even your child's menagerie of stuffed animals needs to be treated. Quarantine the animals by stuffing them in a large, sealed plastic bag and hiding them. The lice should die within 24 hours off the scalp, but it can take 10 days for any eggs to hatch. Leave the animals locked up for at least 2 weeks, just to prevent reinfestation.

- *Repeat treatment.* Keep an eye out for new nits, especially 1–2 weeks after the initial treatment. If more lice appear, repeat the treatment.

- *Sometimes it's not nice to share.* Teach your child not to share combs, brushes, hats, scarves, hair barrettes, and other personal items that go on the head. Try to explain how the lice travel from head to head, and give your child his own hair supplies so he won't feel the need to borrow from a friend.

- *Spread the word.* Once you spot a louse, notify school officials, camp counselors, and day-care workers to prevent it from spreading to other children. All it takes is one louse to louse up the scalps of all the other kids your child plays with.

Natural Remedies

All of the natural remedies listed below can be used to supplement conventional medical treatment.

Herbal
Use one or more of the remedies listed below. Dosage varies according to age; see the chart on page 25 to determine the correct dose for your child.

- Garlic has antiparasitic properties and can help ward off a lice infestation. Give your child 1 dose, 3 times daily, for 5 days.
- Prepare a strong goldenseal tea and wash your child's scalp with it once a day.
- Tea tree oil is a disinfectant that not only is effective in healing the skin but it also can help get rid of head lice. Add 25–30 drops of Tea tree oil to 1 pint of water and rub the mixture on your child's scalp 2 or 3 times daily. After moistening the hair, remove lice and nits using a fine-toothed comb.

An Ounce of Prevention

You can teach your child not to share combs and brushes or to wear other people's hats, but that's not always enough to avoid a lice invasion. Once your child brings these nasty little creatures home, however, you can stop their spread by treating the problem right away, and washing your child's clothes, bed linens and towels separately in very hot water. If possible, do not allow your child to put his head on couches, chairs and other household furniture (except, of course, his bed). You don't want your child to feel unwelcome or unloved, but lice will spread to other family members if given a chance.

When to Call for Help

Most lice infestations can be wiped out with a simple round of over-the-counter treatments. However, check with your doctor before treating children under the age of 2, if you are pregnant or nursing, or if either one of you has sensitive skin, allergies, or asthma. You'll want to talk to your doctor if the lice have spread to the eyebrows and eyelashes, since a milder treatment might be needed.

Marine Stings

An afternoon at the beach frolicking in the waves and building sand castles can be fun for the entire family. That is, until you hear a piercing scream that follows a sting or poke from a jellyfish, Portuguese man-of-war, sea urchin, coral, or other ocean creature.

Jellyfish and Portuguese man-of-wars float at the surface of the water, dragging long, stinging tentacles behind them as they wait patiently for a bit of food to wander within reach. If your child falls into the grasp of one of these annoying creatures, a nasty sting may be the result. And your child is not necessarily safe on land: These clear, bubble-like creatures and their broken off bits of tentacle can keep on stinging for several days after they've washed up on shore.

Other animals, such as sea urchins and coral, don't sting, but can puncture or cut the skin and release venom if your child tries to mess with them. Anything other than a superficial sting or bite should be seen by a doctor to minimize the risk of infection. You can, however, treat minor marine stings on your own.

Traditional Treatments

Dealing with the stingers of the sea. If your child encounters a jellyfish or Portuguese man-of-war, get him out of the water as soon as possible to assess the condition and extent of the injuries. The tentacles of both creatures consist of tiny spikes that release toxins into the skin. These invisible stingers remain in the skin until they are removed, but they can be scraped off, using a credit card or a piece of cardboard to do the job.

Next, rinse the area with salt water. (Fresh water can make the situation worse by causing the remaining stingers to pump out more venom.) Then neutralize the stingers with a paste made by mixing a tablespoon of meat tenderizer with a few drops of rubbing alcohol. Apply the mixture directly to the stings and leave it on for 15–20 minutes. To treat the pain and inflammation, give your child acetaminophen; follow package directions for dosage information.

Coping with ocean cuts and puncture wounds. Stepping on or scraping against coral or sea urchins can cause cuts and potentially serious puncture wounds. First remove the spines or bits of coral by gently brushing off the area with your hand, then applying a piece of adhesive tape to and removing it from the site. Next, wash the wound thoroughly with soap and water, then soak it in hot water—110–115 degrees F—for a half hour (or longer if your child will hold still). The heat will break down any toxins left at the wound site.

The ocean contains the bacteria that cause tetanus, so be sure your child's vaccinations are up-to-date. Tetanus is included in the series of DTP shots, (Diphtheria, Tetanus, Pertussis), that your child should receive from the pediatrician between the ages of 2 months and 5 years, but a tetanus booster is required every 10 years after that.

Natural Remedies

All of the natural remedies listed below can be used to supplement conventional medical treatment.

Herbal
Use one or more of the remedies listed below.

- Aloe vera gel eases the pain and reduces swelling. Apply fresh gel directly to the wound site.
- Apply a few drops of tea tree oil to the site. No need to dilute it.

An Ounce of Prevention

Before heading off to the beach, teach your child how to spot jellyfish, sea urchins, and other potential hazards from the deep. Tell your child not to touch anything he's uncertain about without talking it over with you first. Dress your child in old tennis shoes or aquatic shoes with rubber soles before he enters the ocean to prevent cuts to the feet.

When to Call for Help

Most marine stings cause pain and swelling, and some may also cause nausea and cramps, but most do not pose serious health risks. However, if your child has any difficulty breathing or tightness of the throat, seek medical help immediately. Your child may be experiencing an allergic reaction to the marine animal's toxins.

If your child winds up with a cut caused by a piece of coral, contact your doctor. Cuts on coral often lead to infections, since the jagged coral can cut deep, in addition to secreting potentially dangerous toxins. Deep puncture wounds, such as those caused by sea urchins or other spiny creatures, should also be seen by a doctor, since these injuries are also prone to infection. Wounds that are more than a ½ inch deep should be seen by a doctor.

Measles

Not long ago, parents considered measles a rite of passage of childhood. Today, this highly infectious disease is relatively rare in the United States because most parents have their children immunized against it. Parents in developing countries where the vaccine isn't available aren't so lucky: Measles kill more than 1 million children worldwide every year.

The measles virus takes hold 7–14 days after a child has been exposed to it. During the first stage of the disease, the child shows symptoms of a common cold—runny nose, cough, inflamed throat, red and watery eyes, and a moderate fever. The measles virus parts ways with the common cold several days later, when tiny, salt-like white spots appear inside the mouth.

Following the white spots, the classic measles rash appears, first on the forehead along the hairline and behind the ears. The rash then spreads down the body, the cough gets worse, and the fever spikes to as high as 105 degrees. The rash, which lasts about a week, is mildly itchy. Your child will be infectious for 5 days after the rash appears.

In a typical case of the measles, a child suffers a week or so of feeling lousy. The real danger comes from secondary infections, such as ear infection, pneumonia, bronchitis or encephalitis (an infection of the lining of the brain). These problems can be tended to in most cases, as long as a child receives appropriate medical care. In addition, the following natural remedies can minimize your child's discomfort during the recovery process.

Traditional Treatments

- *Easy does it.* Since measles is caused by a virus, there's little you can do to speed the course of the disease. Your mission is to keep your child as comfortable as possible. Try a non-aspirin pain reliever to take the edge off the pain and to control the fever. Do not give a child under age 18 aspirin (including "baby aspirin"), which can cause the potentially fatal Reye's syndrome. You may want to use cough medicines and decongestants to ease the respiratory problems, especially if a chronic cough is keeping your child up at night.
- *Cool it.* If your child has a high fever, consider a sponge bath to help bring his temperature down. Add a little cornstarch to the water to calm an itchy rash.
- *Dim the lights.* Sunlight or glare can be disturbing to the light-sensitive eyes of a child with measles. (Never fear, the sensitivity will pass without damage to your child's eyes.) Pull the shades or have your child put on sunglasses if excessive light hurts his eyes.
- *Play misty for me.* Use a cool-mist vaporizer in your child's room to moisten your child's throat and make breathing easier. Be sure to follow the manufacturer's cleaning directions, to avoid growth of mold and bacteria in the water.

Natural Remedies

All of the natural remedies listed below can be used to supplement conventional medical treatment.

Diet and Nutrition

Use one or more of the remedies listed below. Dosage varies according to age; see the chart on pages 14–15 to determine to correct dose for your child. Some vitamins can be used topically, as noted. For good food sources of particular nutrients, see pages 9–13.

- Vitamin A helps heal the tender mucous membranes. Give your child 1 dose a day for 10 days.

- Vitamin C boosts the immune system. Give your child 1 dose 3 times a day.
- Encourage your child to drink as much water as possible to avoid dehydration, which often accompanies high fever.
- Zinc strengthens the immune system and assists in cell repair. Give your child 1 dose a day for up to 10 days.

Herbal

Use one or more of the remedies listed below. Dosage varies according to age; see the chart on page 25 to determine the correct dose for your child.

- Offer your child chamomile tea to help reduce the accompanying fever.
- To reduce the itch, give your child a cool oatmeal bath.
- A combination of echinacea and goldenseal can help clear the infection and soothe the skin. Give your child 1 dose every 3 hours, until fever breaks. (Don't use echinacea for more than 10 days or it will lose its effectiveness.)

Homeopathy

Use one homeopathic treatment at a time, based on your child's specific symptoms. For dosage information, see the chart on pages 31–37. Discontinue use if the symptoms disappear.

- *Belladonna (Atropha belladonna)* 30c or Aconite 30c: Use if your child has a high fever, cold symptoms, or a throbbing headache. Give 1 dose every 2 hours for up to 8 doses.
- *Euphrasia (Euphrasia officinalis)* 6c: Use for high fever, cold symptoms, and red, swollen eyes. Give 1 dose every 2 hours for up to 8 doses.
- *Gelsemium (Gelsemium sempervirens)* 30x or 9c: Use if your child has a fever, sleepy-looking eyes, and runny nose. Give 1 dose every 2 hours for up to 8 doses.
- *Pulsatilla (Pulsatilla nigricans)* 6c: Use for a child with fever but no thirst, light-sensitive eyes, and dry cough (especially at night). Give 1 dose every 2 hours for up to 8 doses.
- *Sulphur* 6c: Use for a child with a purplish rash that is slow to clear. Give 1 dose every 2 hours for up to 8 doses.

An Ounce of Prevention

A measles vaccine is available, so most children should never have to deal with this childhood malady. Have your child immunized at 15 months and again before entering school, or at 10–12 years of age, depending on the advice of your physician. Most children receive the measles vaccine in combination with the mumps and rubella vaccines; the side effects (tenderness at the injection site and low fever) are usually mild. Discuss the matter with your doctor if you are concerned about immunizing your child.

WARNING: Rubella (a type of measles sometimes referred to as German measles) can cause serious birth defects if a woman contracts the disease during the first 4 months of pregnancy. Before becoming pregnant, a woman who has not had the disease (or is not certain whether she has had the vaccine) should have a blood test to confirm immunity. If necessary, she should receive the vaccine.

When to Call the Doctor

A simple case of the measles usually doesn't require medical attention, but the secondary infections it causes can lead to a trip to the doctor. Complications, such as ear infections and pneumonia, are relatively common and need to be treated with antibiotics. Call the doctor if your child pulls on his ear frequently or complains of an earache, or if you spot a yellowish discharge from his eyes or nose. Also keep an eye out for labored breathing, wheezing, and prolonged coughing, which can be symptoms of pneumonia.

In rare cases, more serious complications occur. Call for emergency assistance if your child goes into convulsions, experiences a leg cramp or spasm, or if you can't wake him from a deep sleep.

Mumps

If your child's face puffs up with a case of mumps, there's not much you can do, aside from forbidding your other children from calling him chipmunk cheeks (a surprisingly accurate description of the condition).

Mumps (*parotitis*) is a viral infection of the saliva-producing parotid glands (located in front of each ear) and the submaxillary glands (found beneath the jaw). Symptoms first appear 2–4 weeks after exposure to the virus. (A child is contagious from about 6 days before the onset of illness to 9 or 10 days after the glands have become swollen.)

A case of mumps begins with malaise, headache, muscle ache, fever, and headache. Over the next few days, the salivary glands gradually swell and grow tender. Once the virus takes hold, your child will feel weak, feverish and achy, and your mission will be to keep him as comfortable as possible. After about a week, the swelling will diminish; your child's face should be back to normal within 10 days.

Traditional Treatments

- *Take it easy.* Unfortunately, there's not much you can do once your child comes down with mumps, except relieve the symptoms. For fever and general achiness, give your child acetaminophen or ibuprofen. Never give a child under age 18 aspirin (including "baby aspirin") if you think he has the mumps; the combination of aspirin and a viral infection has been linked to Reye's syndrome.
- *Keep it wet.* Since the saliva-producing parotid glands must work overtime to moisten meals when your child has mumps, offer your child wet foods that will slide right down, such as soup, shakes, gelatin, and puddings.

Natural Remedies

All of the natural remedies listed below can be used to supplement conventional medical treatment.

Diet and Nutrition

Use one or more of the remedies listed below. Dosage varies according to age; see the chart on pages 14–15 to determine to correct dose for your child. For good food sources of particular nutrients, see pages 9–13.

- Avoid acidic drinks, such as fruit juices, which increase the painful flow of saliva.
- Stick to soft foods to minimize pain when chewing and swallowing.
- Beta-carotene can help heal mucous membranes. Give your child 2 doses for 10 days.
- Vitamin C strengthens the immune system. Give your child 1 dose of vitamin C 3 times a day for 1 week.
- Zinc boosts the immune system and promotes healing. Give your child 1 dose twice a day for a week to 10 days.

Herbal

Use one or more of the remedies listed below. Dosage varies according to age; see the chart on page 25 to determine the correct dose for your child.

- Use castor oil compresses to ease the pain of tender, swollen glands. Heat the oil to a warm—not hot—temperature. Soak a clean washcloth in the oil and apply it to the glands for 10 or 15 minutes, 2 or 3 times a day.
- Give a restless child chamomile tea twice a day.
- To relieve a headache, rub peppermint oil onto your child's temples.

Homeopathy

Use one homeopathic treatment at a time, based on your child's specific symptoms. For dosage information, see the chart on pages 31–37. Discontinue use if the symptoms disappear.

- *Aconite (Aconitum napellus)* 30c: Use when symptoms include fever. Give 1 dose every 4 hours for up to 8 doses.
- *Belladonna (Atropha belladonna)* 30c: Use for high fever accompanied by a flushed face. Give 1 dose every 4 hours for up to 10 doses.
- *Pilocarpin mur. (Pilocarpin muriaticum)* 6c: Use if your child's saliva is sticky and thick. Give 1 dose every 4 hours for up to 8 doses.
- *Phytolacca (Phytolacca decandra)* 12x or 6c: Use when the submaxillary glands (beneath the jaw) are swollen and hard or when there is ear pain when swallowing. Give 1 dose every 4 hours for up to 10 doses.
- *Pulsatilla (Pulsatilla nigricans)* 6c: Use for swollen and painful testicles. Give 1 dose every 4 hours for up to 10 doses.

An Ounce of Prevention

The easiest way to prevent mumps is to have your child immunized against the disease. At the age of 15 months, most children receive the MMR vaccine, which covers measles and rubella, as well as mumps. A booster vaccine is given when the child enters school, or at 10–12 years of age, depending on the advice of your physician. The side effects (tenderness at the injection site and low fever) are usually mild. Discuss the matter with your doctor if you are concerned about immunizing your child.

When to Call for Help

Mumps should be diagnosed by your doctor because other diseases can also cause swelling of the glands near the face. Different viral or bacterial infections can lead to swollen lymph nodes, which may look like mumps to the untrained eye. (Lymph nodes swell below the jaw; the parotid glands swell above the jawline.)

In rare cases, mumps may lead to encephalitis (an infection of the brain or spinal cord); call your doctor if your child feels excessively drowsy, complains of a severe headache or stiff neck, or shrinks away from bright light. Male infertility, caused by an infection in the testicles of adolescent boys with mumps, is less common than widely perceived, but call your doctor if your teenage son comes down with the mumps.

Muscle Aches and Cramps

Muscles get taken for granted: Most people give little or no thought to the delicate balance of chemicals, oxygen, and blood required to keep their muscles working efficiently. Subtle imbalances and a buildup of waste material in the muscles can result in not-so-subtle pain and cramping.

Children who exercise or play in extreme heat sometimes get painful daytime cramps in the calf, foot, or abdomen. Other times cramps attack in the middle of the night, ripping your child out of a deep and relaxing sleep. A tough day of play can result in a morning of stiff and achy muscles if your child overdoes it on the playground.

Muscle pains and cramps aren't the exclusive domain of athletes. In fact, less athletic kids can face serious pain when they overdo in gym class or push too hard to keep up with their friends. Whatever the cause, muscles cramps usually ease up in a matter of minutes, but you can ease your child's pain by following a few simple steps.

Traditional Treatments

Stretch it out. It's going to hurt, but stretching and rubbing a muscle in spasm helps to relax the cramping. Don't treat the area roughly, since these tight muscles will tear and strain easily if not handled with care. Massaging the area stimulates blood flow and helps relax the muscle. Press firmly and rub in long, smooth strokes across the entire length of the muscle.

Offer soothing and encouraging words as you work with your child to loosen the area.

Heat it up. After the muscle has been loosened, apply a warm, wet compress or heating pad to the area. This will further increase blood flow and relaxation of the muscle. There is one exception: Muscle cramps that are caused by excessive heat and overexertion should be treated with a cold compress to the affected muscle.

Drink it down. Your child needs to drink plenty of fluids during exercise to minimize the risk of cramping. Encourage your child to drink a few ounces of water or sports drink every 15–20 minutes during active play or exercise.

Take one of these and call me in the morning. You may be able to avoid some nighttime cramping and muscle pain following strenuous exercise by giving your child a dose of acetaminophen before bed. The painkiller can help ease the pain and minimize tissue swelling.

Natural Remedies

All of the natural remedies listed below can be used to supplement conventional medical treatment.

Diet and Nutrition

Use one or more of the remedies mentioned below. Dosage varies according to age; see the chart on pages 14–15 to determine to correct dose for your child. For good food sources of particular nutrients, see pages 9–13.

- Calcium is important for proper muscle contraction. Give your child 1 dose of calcium 3 times a day for 2 or 3 days after an episode of muscle cramping or overexertion.
- Magnesium is important for muscle relaxation. Give your child 1 dose 3 times a day for 2 days after muscle cramping or overexertion.

Herbal

Use one or more of the remedies listed below. Dosage varies according to age; see the chart on page 25 to determine the correct dose for your child.

- Arnica helps relieve muscle cramps and pain resulting from overuse (in addition to being widely used against bruising). Dilute tincture of arnica by mixing 1 tablespoon of tincture with 1 pint of cold water, then soak a clean cloth in the mixture and hold it against the affected muscle. Another option is to use arnica ointments or lotions, which can be applied directly to the skin. (Don't use either topical treatment if the skin is broken.)
- Peppermint tea can help control muscle spasms or cramps. Give your child 1 dose 2–3 times during the day.

Acupressure

Use one or more of the acupressure points listed below. For a diagram showing the specific pressure points, see pages 40–41.

- Middle of a Person (Governing Vessel 26): This point is located two-thirds of the way up from the upper lip to the nose.
- Supporting Mountain (Bladder 57): To find this point, place your fingers in the center of the base of the calf muscle, midway between the crease behind the knee and the heel, at the bottom of the calf muscle bulge.

An Ounce of Prevention

Most muscle aches and cramps can be prevented by warming up and cooling down thoroughly before and after exercise, and by resisting the temptation to do too much exercise, too quickly. Encourage your child to get regular exercise, but to pace himself and build intensity gradually.

In addition, remind your child to drink plenty of water during exercise or play to minimize the risk of cramping. A diet rich in calcium and magnesium can also help prevent cramps, especially those that strike at night.

When to Call for Help

Most muscle aches and cramps clear up within minutes, and they very rarely demand medical attention. However, you should call your physician if the problem lasts more than 10 or 15 minutes, if cramping becomes a chronic problem, or if the muscle pain is accompanied by fever, loss of strength in the muscles, swollen or enlarged joints, or a rash.

Nosebleeds

Nosebleeds almost always look worse than they really are. The sight of blood can unnerve the bravest of kids (and parents), though most nosebleeds are nothing to worry about.

Nosebleeds are among the most common bleeding emergencies involving children, affecting more than half of all children between the ages of 6 and 10. Nosebleeds can be caused by trauma to the nose (from an elbow to the face during an outbreak of roughhousing), minor cuts or scratches to the delicate nasal passages (from picking the nose using a sharp fingernail), or vigorous nose-blowing (such as occurs during a bout with the flu). Arid, hot air can also dry out the mucous membranes, causing irritation and nosebleeds.

Noses have a tendency to bleed because the lining of the nasal passage is replete with tiny blood vessels and small capillaries. Once broken, these vessels will bleed until a clot forms to block the flow of blood. Fortunately, most broken vessels in the nose clot readily, within 10 minutes or so.

Traditional Treatments

Take a deep breath. If you have nasal spray decongestant in the medicine cabinet, now is the time to pull it out and give your child a nostril full. These over-the-counter products shrink the blood vessels and encourage the formation of scabs.

The firm squeeze. Start by asking your child to give one strong blow of the nose to clear any partial clots and mucus. Have your child breathe through his mouth, then gently but firmly squeeze the nostrils together, holding a tissue or clean washcloth over the nose. Hold the nostril shut for 10–15 minutes, which should be enough time to allow the blood to clot and stop the bleeding.

Sit up straight. Have your child sit up in your lap or sit straight in a chair while squeezing the nostrils. Reclining will only cause the blood to flow down the back of the throat, which is guaranteed to taste bad and may also cause an upset stomach.

Don't just squeeze, freeze. A cold compress against the nose will help constrict the blood vessels and slow the blood flow. Soak a clean cloth in cold water or wrap ice in a cloth and apply it to the affected area. (Don't apply ice directly to the skin or it can cause frostbite.)

Natural Remedies

All of the natural remedies listed below can be used to supplement conventional medical treatment.

Diet and Nutrition

Dosage varies according to age; see the chart on pages 14–15 to determine to correct dose for your child. Some vitamins can be used topically, as noted. For good food sources of particular nutrients, see pages 9–13.

- A thin layer of vitamin E oil can be applied to the nasal passage to keep the nose moist, if your child's nose is dry and irritated. (Nonpetroleum jelly can also be used.)
- Vitamin K helps the blood clot. If your child experiences frequent nosebleeds, give him 10 micrograms of vitamin K 3 times a day for 2 weeks.

Homeopathy

Use one homeopathic treatment at a time, based on your child's specific symptoms. For dosage information, see the chart on pages 31–37. Discontinue use if the symptoms disappear.

- *Arnica (Arnica montana)* 6c: Use if your child develops a nosebleed following an injury. Give 1 dose every 2 minutes for up to 10 doses.
- *Ipecac. (Cephaelis ipecacuanha)* 6c: Use if the blood is bright red. Give 1 dose every 2 minutes for up to 10 doses.
- *Phosphorus* 6c: Use if the nosebleed is caused by excessive nose-blowing. Give 1 dose every 2 minutes for up to 10 doses.

Acupressure

Use one or more of the acupressure points listed below. For a diagram showing the specific pressure points, see pages 40–41.

- Eyes Bright (Bladder 1): This point is located in the hollow at the inner corner of the eye just above the tear duct.
- Facial Beauty (Stomach 3): To find this point, place your fingers at the bottom of the cheekbone, directly below the pupil of the eye.
- Joining the Valley (Large Intestine 4): Apply steady pressure on the point in the webbing between the thumb and index finger at the highest spot of the muscle when the thumb and index finger are brought closest together.
- Middle of a Person (Governing Vessel 26): This point is located two-thirds of the way up from the upper lip to the nose.

An Ounce of Prevention

Nosebleeds caused by trauma or injury cannot always be prevented, but many chronic episodes can be prevented by keeping the noise moist and clean. Nose-picking can cause nosebleeds, so discourage the practice among your children. To prevent dried-out nasal passages, run a vaporizer or humidifier in your child's bedroom, especially in the winter and at night. (Clean the appliance regularly, following the manufacturer's directions.)

If your child has a nosebleed, you can prevent a recurrence by discouraging your child from blowing his nose after a nosebleed, except for that initial blow to clear the nose before holding the nose to form a clot. (Forceful blowing after the clot has formed can disrupt the scab and cause the bleeding to start up all over again.) Likewise, tell your child to avoid strenuous play, especially involving activities like gymnastics or hanging upside down, which can put pressure on the nasal passages. Remember, it takes 7–10 days to recover fully from a severe nosebleed.

When to Call for Help

Most nosebleeds make a mess but don't pose any serious medical threat. However, you should contact a doctor if your child has a history of bleeding or clotting problems, if the bleeding continues after 15 minutes, if your child experiences difficulty breathing, or if the nosebleed follows a blow to the head. Also, if your child experiences nosebleeds more than once a month, contact your pediatrician to rule out a more dangerous condition, such as high blood pressure or hemophilia.

Pinkeye

It usually strikes first thing in the morning: Your child wakes up and you notice that his eyes are pink and swollen, or worse yet, "glued" shut with a thick crust of yellowish discharge. Good morning, pinkeye.

Pinkeye (*conjunctivitis*) is an infection of the lining of the membrane inside the eyelid that can be caused by both bacteria and cold viruses. (Though the causes may be different, the symptoms are the same for both types of pinkeye.) The condition often accompanies a cold, and is common in small children who touch everything in reach, then rub their eyes at nap-time. Other eye problems can be caused by allergies, irritants, or minor injuries. Sand, dirt, or a wayward gnat that lands in your child's eye can all stir up trouble.

The viral form of pinkeye runs its course and disappears within a week or so, just as a cold would. Bacterial infections may refuse to depart without the use of antibiotic drops or ointments. If your child's condition does not improve within 5 days or so, contact your child's pediatrician, who can prescribe antibiotics.

The condition is certainly uncomfortable, but it's not usually serious, except in newborns. Pinkeye is highly contagious, however, and can easily be passed from one eye to the other, or one child to another. Explain to your child the importance of not touching the infected eye, and washing his hands frequently to avoid spreading the disease.

Traditional Treatments

- *Close your eyes, and relax.* The best way to soothe your child's eyes is to apply warm compresses with the eyes closed. Use a clean washcloth or rag; when it cools warm it up and do it again. Try to apply compresses for 5–10 minutes, at least 3 times a day. The more often you do this, the better, since the microorganisms that cause pinkeye can't tolerate heat.
- *Open your eyes.* Pinkeye can cause the eyes to ooze and crust over during the night. Comfort your child (it can be quite upsetting to wake up and find your eyes glued shut), then use a warm compress to "unstick" your child's gloppy eyes.
- *Don't make contact.* If your child is old enough to wear contact lenses, tell him to remove them when the pinkeye first shows up. The lenses can irritate the cornea when pinkeye is present.
- *Good from the first drop.* Sterile saline drops can soothe infected eyes, if your child is willing to cooperate long

enough to allow you to put in the drops. The best technique: Have your child look at the ceiling, then pull down your child's lower eyelid and place a drop of liquid under the eye. Be careful not to let the dropper touch the eye or the surrounding area, since the bacteria may spread to the saline solution.

- *Don't get the red out.* Skip the over-the-counter eye drops designed to reduce redness. These drops will do nothing to fight infection and if used for more than a couple of days, products containing the active ingredient tetrahydrozoline can cause "rebound" eye vessel dilation, which will actually increase the redness.
- *Keep an eye out.* Covering the infected eye with a patch or gauze pad creates a nice warm, dark breeding ground for bacteria. The patch also inhibits the eye's natural cleansing system, tears, because your child will be unable to blink with a patch on his eye.
- *Doctor's orders.* If you don't see any improvement in 5–7 days, seek medical attention. Your child's doctor may prescribe an antibiotic eye ointment or eye drops to fight bacterial infection.

Natural Remedies

All of the natural remedies listed below can be used to supplement conventional medical treatment.

Diet and Nutrition

Use one or more of the remedies listed below. Dosage varies according to age; see the chart on pages 14–15 to determine to correct dose for your child. Some vitamins can be used topically, as noted. For good food sources of particular nutrients, see pages 9–13.

- Vitamin A promotes healthy eyes and boosts the immune system. Give your child half a dose twice a day for 3 days.
- Vitamin C reduces inflammation and promotes healing. Give your child 1 dose of vitamin C twice a day for a week. Also

encourage your child to eat a diet rich in green and yellow fruits and vegetables.

- Zinc can work wonders on eye disorders, in addition to boosting the immune system's infection-fighting power. Give your child ½ a dose twice a day for 5 days.

Herbal

- Make a warm compress of eyebright tea. Eyebright helps clear eye infections by increasing blood flow to the eye, which helps to wash away the crust from the eye. Simmer 1 teaspoon of the dried herb in 1 pint of water for 10 minutes. When the tea is warm, not hot, moisten a washcloth or clean rag and place the compress on your child's eyes for 5–10 minutes. Repeat 3 or 4 times a day, if possible.

Homeopathy

Use one homeopathic treatment at a time, based on your child's specific symptoms. For dosage information, see the chart on pages 31–37. Discontinue use if the symptoms disappear.

- *Aconite (Aconitum napellus)* 30c: Use if pinkeye appears during a cold. Give 1 dose every hour for up to 8 doses.
- *Argentum nit. (Argentum nitricum)* 6c: Use if the infection includes a lot of discharge, which can range from runny to thick. Give 1 dose every hour for up to 8 doses.
- *Pulsatilla (Pulsatilla nigricans)* 12x or 6c: Use if the infection includes thick, yellow discharge. Give 1 dose twice daily for 2 days.

Acupressure

Use one or more of the acupressure points listed below. For a diagram showing the specific pressure points, see pages 40–41.

- Bigger Rushing (Liver 3): This point is located on the top of the foot in the valley between the big toe and the second toe.

- Eyes Bright (Bladder 1): To find this point, place your fingers in the hollow at the inner corner of the eye, just above the tear ducts.

An Ounce of Prevention

Pinkeye spreads easily, so your mission is to teach your child to practice good hygiene:

- Tell your child never to use anyone else's washcloth or face towels.
- Encourage your child to wash his hands before and after touching his eyes.

In addition, if someone in the household comes down with pinkeye, wash that person's towels, pillowcases, and other linens separately and with plenty of detergent, in hot water, to prevent further spread of the infection. After you load the washer, scrub your hands with antibacterial soap to kill any microorganisms that might be on your hands.

Avoid exposing your child to smoke, toxic fumes, chlorinated water and other eye irritants as much as possible.

When to Call for Help

Pinkeye can usually be treated at home; however, you should call your doctor if the infection does not clear up (or gets worse) after 5 days or if there is a green discharge from the eye or the eye looks cloudy (these could be symptoms of a herpes infection in the eye, a condition that can cause blindness).

In addition, call the doctor if your child reports any vision problems or light sensitivity (including seeing halos around lights), or if you notice any irregularities in the size of your child's pupils. If your child is less than a year old, *always* call the doctor at the first sign of any eye infection.

Pinworms

The thought is sometimes worse than the reality. Many parents become quite distressed when they learn that their children have worms, but the condition is rarely serious and always easily cured.

Pinworms (*Enterobius vermicularis*) are a common type of intestinal roundworm that live in humans and apes, spread from hand to mouth. They look like thin, white threads, about ¼ to ½ inch long. During the night or early in the morning, the female worms crawl out of the large intestine to the anus, where they deposit their microscopic eggs. The eggs cause itching and irritation, so when the child scratches the area, he traps the eggs on his hands and under his fingernails. If the child does not thoroughly scrub his hands and fingernails before he touches his fingers to his mouth, the eggs enter the digestive system where they are hatched, and the cycle repeats itself.

These nasty little creatures rapidly spread from one child to another—or from one family member to another—because the eggs also attach themselves to other objects the child might touch, including clothing, toys, and food. An estimated 10–30 percent of American children come down with pinworms before they reach adulthood.

The worms will live and reproduce in your child's digestive system until the cycle is broken through medical intervention. If your child complains about an itchy bottom, or you notice him scratching, take steps to control the problem before it spreads to other family members. The following suggestions can help.

Traditional Treatments

- *How about 'good morning' first?* The best way to confirm the pinworm diagnosis is to gather the eggs yourself. First thing in the morning, ask your child to lay quietly while you search the area, using a piece of tape to collect the evidence. Wash your hands thoroughly, then bring the tape to the doctor for his inspection.
- *Fill that prescription.* Your pediatrician will prescribe a medication that eradicates the worms. The drug prevents them from metabolizing the sugars they need to survive. One dose is usually all it take to get rid of them. A follow-up treatment may be necessary if the worms have been passed back and forth between other family members.
- *Try a soothing wipe.* If your child's bottom itches, moisten a disposable rag with water or use diaper wipes to clean the area thoroughly. Be sure to dispose of the dirty rag or wipe when finished.
- *Did you wash your hands?* Good hand-washing habits must be enforced to prevent reinfection. Let your child pick out a favorite type of soap and encourage him to use it.
- *No place to hide.* Cut your child's fingernails, and keep them short. Make it tough on the eggs to hitch a ride. Short nails will also prevent your child from hurting himself if he can't keep from scratching.
- *One for all, and all for one.* Pinworms don't discriminate based on age or sex; they'll feast on anyone who lets them. When one family member gets infected, there's a good chance the infection will spread, so treatment should involve the entire family.

Natural Remedies

All of the natural remedies listed below can be used to supplement conventional medical treatment.

Diet and Nutrition

- Pinworms feast on refined carbohydrates and simple sugars, such as cookies and candies. Limit these foods in your child's diet while adding more high-fiber grains and raw vegetables, to assist in getting rid of the creatures.

Herbal
Use one or more of the remedies listed below. Dosage varies according to age; see the chart on page 25 to determine the correct dose for your child.

- Garlic is an effective antiparasitic agent. Give your child 1–2 doses of odorless garlic twice daily, for 2 weeks.
- Wormwood is another antiparasitic herb that can be effective in the treatment of pinworms. Give your child 1 dose, twice daily, for up to 1 week.

Homeopathy
For dosage information, see the chart on pages 31–37. Discontinue use if the symptoms disappear.

- *Cina (Cina artemisia maritima)* 12x or 6c: Use if your child has an itchy bottom. Give 1 dose twice daily for 5–7 days.

An Ounce of Prevention

Start by teaching your child to wash his hands after going to the bathroom and before eating. To the degree you can, try to break oral habits, such as thumb-sucking, fingernail-biting, and putting every object within reach into the mouth. If pinworms show up in your household, take prompt action by following the steps listed above to prevent them from spreading to other family members.

When to Call for Help

You can't take care of this one on your own. Call your doctor to get the necessary medication to clear up the problem. With medication, the condition should clear within a couple of days. However, after the initial treatment you should remain on the lookout for recurrence during the next 2 weeks or so, since your child can be reinfected though a second exposure to the worms from another family member or friend with the problem.

In rare cases, the worm can enter and irritate the vagina. Notify your doctor immediately if your little girl with pinworms complains of vaginal pain, itching, or discharge.

Poison Ivy, Oak, and Sumac

One night your child goes to bed smooth-skinned and blemish-free. The following morning, his arms and legs are covered with red, itchy blisters. Remember that walk in the park yesterday? Remember those plants with the telltale three leaves?

Poison ivy, poison oak, and poison sumac all threaten to cause skin reactions in people who come into contact with the leaves, stems, and roots of each of these types of plant. (They contain an oil, urushiol, which acts as a skin irritant to many.) If you have more than one child, one may break out while the other remains clear-skinned—even if they've both been exposed. Many children under the age of 7 have not yet developed a sensitivity to the oil; it takes at least one exposure to develop the allergy that causes the telltale reaction. And some fortunate folks never develop the allergy and can handle the plants without ill effect.

In most cases, red, itchy patches show up 12–48 hours after exposure, when the body rushes histamines and antibodies to the skin to fight the invaders. A few days later, blisters appear, then the oozing and crusting begins. It usually takes 1 to

2 weeks for the itching to fade, and the skin to return to normal.

Once your child develops a rash after exposure to poison ivy, oak, or sumac, all you can do is try to ease the itching, and soothe the sore spots.

Traditional Treatments

If it itches . . . Try to make it stop. Scratching the sores can cause infection and scarring. Try melting an ice cube on the itchy spot, or coat it with calamine lotion or hydrocortisone cream. Another option is to soak your child in a warm bath with either a half cup of baking soda, or colloidal oatmeal added to relieve the itching. (Oatmeal baths, such as Aveeno, are available at most drugstores.)

Consider antihistamines. Over-the-counter antihistamines help relieve itching. And, as an added bonus, they also make many children drowsy, which can help your child snooze until morning without being awakened in an itching frenzy. For proper use, follow dosage information on the package.

Don't make a bad situation worse. Don't apply topical antihistamines or anesthetics, since these products can cause skin rashes in children. Your child has enough irritation to contend with without adding to his burden.

Don't worry about spreading the rash. Don't blame the oozing blisters for spreading the rash. The blisters and irritation show up only where the urushiol touched the skin. It *appears* that the blisters cause the rash to spread because the blisters form gradually over the course of about a week. In fact, what's happening is that the sites exposed to the highest concentrations of urushiol blister first, and those with lower exposures blister a few days later. The sooner your child washes with soap and water after exposure, the milder the outbreak will be.

Natural Remedies

All of the natural remedies listed below can be used to supplement conventional medical treatment.

Diet and Nutrition
Dosage varies according to age; see the chart on pages 14–15 to determine the correct dose for your child. For good food sources of particular nutrients, see pages 9–13.

- Vitamin C reduces inflammation. Give your child 1 dose 2 or 3 times a day for 10 days.

Herbal
Use one or more of the remedies listed below.

- Aloe vera eases the itch and irritation of the rash. Apply the gel from the plant directly to your child's blisters 3 or 4 times a day, as long as necessary. Commercial preparations are also available.
- Jewelweed (*Impatiens biflora*) is nature's remedy for poison ivy. In fact, the plant, which has tiny, orange-yellow flowers and grows 12–18 inches tall, often grows next to the poison ivy plant. If your child is exposed to poison ivy, pick some jewelweed leaves, crush them in your hands, and wipe the plant against your child's skin where it came into contact with the poison ivy. This can help prevent skin irritations. The same topical treatment helps speed the recovery once the rash develops. Commercial preparations are also available.
- The milkweed plant can speed the healing of the rash. Break the stem of the plant and drop the milky juice directly over the rash. Commercial preparations are also available.

Homeopathy
For dosage information, see the chart on pages 31–37. Discontinue use if the symptoms disappear.

- *Rhus tox. (Rhus toxicodendron)* 12x or 6c: Use when your child develops a rash; the remedy helps blisters and prevents spreading. Give 1 dose 3–4 times daily for up to 3 days.

Acupressure
Use one or more of the acupressure points listed below. For a diagram showing the specific pressure points, see pages 40–41.

- Crooked Pond (Large Intestine 11): This point is located on the forearm at the outer edge of the elbow crease.
- Great Abyss (Lung 9): To find this point, place your fingers in the groove at the wrist fold below the base of the thumb.
- Joining the Valley (Large Intestine 4): Apply steady pressure to the point in the webbing between the thumb and index finger. On the outside of the hand, find the highest spot of the muscle where the thumb and index fingers are brought closest together.

An Ounce of Prevention

By far the best way to prevent poison ivy, oak, and sumac rashes is to avoid coming in contact with them. Go to the library and check out a book on poisonous plants and teach your children how to identify the offenders. (Also see the box on page 236.)

If your child is going to be hiking in the woods, consider slathering his legs with a barrier cream to prevent (or minimize) exposure. Products such as Ivy Block or Ivy Shield are available in outdoor sporting goods stores, but they can trap body heat, so use them only when you suspect your child will be exposed. Of course, there are no guarantees that you'll cover every inch of skin, but this method may prevent a major outbreak.

If the family dog joins in on the hike, give him a bath when you get back. The dog won't develop a rash, since the oil is on the surface of his fur, but when your child pets the dog, he will be exposed to the oil-coated fur.

Always have your child wash thoroughly with soap and water after returning from a site that may have had poisonous plants. Of course, the faster you can remove the oil, the greater the likelihood of avoiding an itchy breakout. Wash all clothing and towels afterward in hot water. (Wash garden gloves and tools after using them around these plants, since the oil can remain active for months or years away from the plant.)

WARNING: Never burn yard debris, unless you know there are no poisonous plants mixed in. Inhaling fumes from poison ivy, oak, or sumac can cause a potentially fatal outbreak of blisters and a rash in the mouth, throat, and lungs.

Pick Your Poison

- *Poison ivy*: Remember the adage "Leaves of three, let it be." This three-leafed plant grows as a shrub, a ground cover, or a climbing vine, and thrives in shady areas. It grows throughout the United States, but primarily east of the Rocky Mountains. From region to region, the leaves vary in size, shape, and color; the plant often has white flowers in the spring and white berries in the fall.
- *Poison oak*: Like poison ivy, this plant also has three leaves, but the leaves are the classic oak shape. This plant thrives in the West and Southwest, especially California and Oregon.
- *Poison sumac*: This plant grows as a tall shrub in swamps and wetlands in the Southeast. The plant has white berries and bright green, pointed leaves, configured with 6–10 leaflets opposite each other, with a single leaflet at the end of the stem.

When to Call for Help

Most kids who break out from poison ivy, oak, or sumac feel irritable and itchy for a few days, but that's about the extent of the problem. However, about 15 percent of kids who respond to urushiol experience potentially life-threatening swelling and need emergency treatment with corticosteroids. Call the doctor immediately if your child experiences swelling—either at the rash site or all over the body—4–12 hours after exposure, if your child experiences difficulty breathing, or if the swelling is so severe that your child's eyes swell shut.

Prickly Heat

Prickly heat is your child's body's way of saying, "I'm hot" long before he utters his first word. The itchy, red rash (properly known as *miliaria*) may appear when your little one becomes overheated and sweats. Because children have undeveloped sweat glands that aren't very good at regulating body temperature, sweat can become trapped by blocked or inflamed glands. Instead of reaching the surface of the skin the moisture is trapped in small, blister-like bumps, which may be itchy.

The prickly heat rash usually shows up on the face, neck, shoulders, and in the creases of the elbows, knees and groin, where the sweat glands are most numerous. Older kids can develop prickly heat, too, but they usually have no trouble complaining when they're hot—or taking their clothes off without your assistance.

The rash usually occurs on hot, humid days, but it can also appear in the dead of winter, if your child is overdressed and overheated. The rash usually disappears on its own within a day or two, but the following suggestions can help you comfort your child and speed his recovery.

Traditional Treatments

- *Chill out.* Your first mission is to cool your kid down. Seek refuge in an air-conditioned area, remove several layers of

clothing, or consider giving your child a tepid bath.
- *Don't make a bad situation worse.* Avoid using cornstarch powder or perfumed lotions, which can aggravate the rash. Baby powder can help keep your little one dry, but use it sparingly to avoid too much "dust," which can irritate the lungs.
- *Ease the itch.* If itching is a problem, soak your child in a tepid bath containing baking soda or an oatmeal product, such as Aveeno. If the water doesn't take the edge off the itch, the baking soda or oatmeal might. If a bath seems too ambitious, consider a cool baking soda and water compress for 10 minutes (or as long as your child will tolerate it).
- *"I'm still itchy."* If nothing else seems to work, give your child an over-the-counter, itch-easing antihistamine such as Benadryl Elixir. Follow the package directions for appropriate dosage.

Natural Remedies

All of the natural remedies listed below can be used to supplement conventional medical treatment.

Diet and Nutrition
Use one or more of the remedies listed below. Some vitamins can be used topically, as noted.

- If your child has prickly heat, avoid greasy or spicy foods, which can aggravate the rash.
- Mix 2 tablespoons of powdered vitamin C with ½ cup of aloe vera gel and apply to the rash twice a day to promote healing and soothe the skin.

Herbal
Use one or more of the remedies listed below.

- To take the sting out and hasten healing, apply calendula gel to the rash.
- Spray the rash with this soothing mixture: ½ tablespoon zinc oxide powder, 1 teaspoon baking soda, ½ tablespoon glyc-

erin, ¼ cup rubbing alcohol, ¼ cup witch hazel, and ½ cup rose water. Shake well before using. (You can buy the ingredients at any drugstore.)

Homeopathy
For dosage information, see the chart on pages 31–37. Discontinue use if the symptoms disappear.

• *Apis (Apis mellifica)* 30x or 9c: Use if the rash is red and swollen. Give 1 dose 3 times a day for 2 days.

Acupressure
Use one or more of the acupressure points listed below. For a diagram showing the specific pressure points, see pages 40–41.

• Crooked Pond (Large Intestine 11): This point is located on the forearm at the outer edge of the elbow crease.
• Great Abyss (Lung 9): To find this point, place your fingers in the groove at the wrist fold below the base of the thumb.
• Joining the Valley (Large Intestine 4): Apply steady pressure on the point in the outside webbing between the thumb and index finger, at the highest spot of the muscle when the thumb and index fingers are brought closest together.

An Ounce of Prevention

In most cases, prickly heat can be avoided by keeping your child cool and comfortable. Dress your child in layers, preferably consisting of clothes made of natural fibers that "breathe." Prickly heat occurs in all seasons, so by dressing your child in layers, you can remove clothing as necessary to maintain an appropriate body temperature.

While it's critical that your child wear sunscreen when playing outside, avoid thick, oily products that can clog the sweat glands and cause prickly heat, even in older children. Stick to formulas designed for children.

When to Call for Help

The red, swollen bumps of prickly heat rash should disappear after a couple of days. If the rash persists or you spot signs of infection—a fever, a discharge of pus, red streaks around the inflamed area—contact your doctor. Your child could have introduced bacteria to the area by scratching the itchy patch with dirty fingernails.

Ringworm

The term "ringworm" is really a misnomer; the condition has nothing to do with worms. Instead, it is a fungus that grows on the scalp or skin, starting as a dry, flaky area, then spreading into a circular pattern with a red border that often feels itchy. Scalp ringworm often looks like severe dandruff, but it's accompanied by hair loss.

Ringworm is caused by the same fungus (*tinea*) that causes athlete's foot and jock itch. It is very contagious. Children spread it to one another, and they can also get it from infected dogs and cats.

If your child develops ringworm, visit your doctor to begin treatment before the fungus spreads. Your doctor will probably prescribe an antifungal drug such as *griseofulvin* or *ketoconazole*, but there are other steps you can take to deal with the problem at home.

Traditional Treatments

• *Hands off.* Ringworm can be spread by touching contaminated objects, including brushes, combs, hats, or other objects that come in contact with the hair or skin. If your child has ringworm, keep his personal objects separate from the rest of the family's and from his friends' belongings at school.

- *Call the school.* Tell your child's teacher or day care provider that your child has ringworm, and explain what precautions should be taken to halt the spread of the disease. Basically, your child can do anything he wants, provided the other children don't touch the affected area, or borrow personal items that might carry the fungus. Ask the teacher to discuss the problem with the children, and to try to do this in a way that won't make your child feel singled out for ridicule by explaining that any child can develop the problem.

- *Don't worry, it'll grow back.* Children with scalp ringworm often lose patches of hair. Unless your child has an allergic reaction to the fungus (which isn't common), the hair loss should be temporary. If you notice oozing spots on your child's scalp, see your doctor. He can treat the problem and avoid the scarring that might cause a bald spot. The sooner you act, the less likely your child's scalp will suffer any long-term side effects.

- *Wash your hair, doctor's orders.* If your child has scalp ringworm, his doctor will probably prescribe a medicated shampoo containing the antifungal selenium sulfide. Some over-the-counter products do contain the same active ingredient, but at a lower concentration. Opt for the high-power suds to kill those fungus spores quickly.

- *Hats off.* Not in this case . . . If your child's scalp looks patchy, buy him a special baseball cap and ask his teacher to indulge him by allowing him to wear it at school. Ringworm is nothing to be embarrassed about, but it's often tough convincing a child of that.

- *Slather on the ointment.* If your child has body ringworm, his doctor will prescribe a topical antifungal ointment. In about a week or so, the red, irritated areas should begin to fade. Again, there are over-the-counter ointments that contain the same active ingredients, but you should get faster results by using the stronger treatments prescribed by the doctor. Continue using the product until the last red patches disappear.

Natural Remedies

All of the natural remedies listed below can be used to supplement conventional medical treatment.

Herbal
Use one or more of the remedies listed below.

- Balsam of Peru is an antifungal liquid that can be applied to the affected area. Apply 3 times a day for 2 or 3 weeks.
- Tea tree oil is a strong antifungal herb that can help fight ringworm and other skin infections. Soak a clean washcloth in a mixture of 7–8 drops of tea tree oil and 1 cup of warm water. Apply the compress to the affected area for 10–15 minutes 3 times a day, until the rash disappears. Discard the rag after using.

Homeopathy
Use one homeopathic treatment at a time, based on your child's specific symptoms. For dosage information, see the chart on pages 31–37. Discontinue use if the symptoms disappear.

- *Sulphur* 6c: Use if your child's scalp is infected. Give 1 dose every 4 hours for up to 8 doses.
- *Tellurium* 6c: Use if the ringworm is located on the trunk of your child's body. Give 1 dose every 4 hours for up to 8 doses.

An Ounce of Prevention

You can't stop your child from playing with other children, but you can stop him from playing with a dog or cat infected with ringworm. The disease afflicts dogs and cats as well as humans, and it spreads easily from beast to child. Warn your child to stay away from animals he doesn't know, and to keep an eye out for patches of hair loss, or the characteristic ring, on the family pet. If a pet develops ringworm, go to the veterinarian and have the condition treated promptly to avoid allowing the infection to spread to your children.

When to Call for Help

Ringworm isn't usually serious, but in some cases it may spread quickly and require a doctor's prompt attention. Call your pediatrician to begin treatment as soon as you suspect your child has ringworm. In addition, be on the lookout for signs of infected patches on the skin including high fever, swollen glands, and red streaks around the site.

Roseola

At first you notice your child feels a little warm. Next time you touch him, he feels warmer still. You take his temperature, but each time you reach for the thermometer, it seems his temperature climbs, up to as high as 105 degrees. Then, after several days of high fever, his temperature drops, his lymph glands swell, and a pink rash appears on his stomach and back, then spreads to his arms and neck (it rarely reaches the legs or face). Diagnosis: Roseola.

Roseola (*roseola infantum*) is a viral infection that commonly strikes children between the ages of 6 months and 3 years. It is rare in preschoolers and older children, and does not affect adults. The fever typically lasts between 1 and 4 days, and the rash lingers for 2–4 days.

The virus can be spread to other young children via respiratory contact. The incubation period for the virus is 10 days–2 weeks, and your child remains contagious for 5 days after the fever disappears. As soon as you notice any symptoms, your child should avoid contact with other children, especially those under age 3, who are most susceptible. The disease can resolve itself quickly or drag on for about a week. Most cases of roseola are mild, but there is a possibility the high fever may trigger convulsions, which would require immediate medical attention.

Traditional Treatments

- *This too shall pass.* Treatment for roseola involves lowering the fever, and keeping the child comfortable while the disease runs its course. Use acetaminophen or ibuprofen to lower the fever, and ease the pain and aches. (Do not give aspirin or "baby aspirin" to a child under age 18; the combination of aspirin and a viral infection has been linked to the development of Reye's syndrome, a potentially life-threatening disease.)
- *Drink up.* Be sure your child drinks plenty of fluids. The high fever associated with roseola can cause dehydration.

Natural Remedies

All of the natural remedies listed below can be used to supplement conventional medical treatment.

Diet and Nutrition

Dosage varies according to age; see the chart on pages 14–15 to determine to correct dose for your child. For good food sources of particular nutrients, see pages 9–13.

- Vitamin C helps reduce inflammation and calm a fever. Give your child 1 dose, 3 times a day until the fever breaks.

Herbal

Use one or more of the remedies listed below. Dosage varies according to age; see the chart on page 25 to determine the correct dose for your child.

- Echinacea and goldenseal are known for their antibacterial and antiviral properties. Give your child 1 dose of combination formula every 2 hours, until the fever breaks.
- If your child is bothered by an itchy rash, give him a soothing oatmeal bath.

Homeopathy

Use one homeopathic treatment at a time, based on your child's specific symptoms. For dosage information, see the chart on pages 31–37. Discontinue use if the symptoms disappear.

- *Belladonna (Atropha belladonna)* 200x or 15c: Use if your child develops a high fever and tender glands in the neck below the jaw. Give 1 dose every 4 hours for up to 8 doses.
- *Phytolacca (Phytolacca decandra)* 12x or 6c: Use if your child develops swollen glands and has difficulty swallowing. Give 1 dose every 4 hours for up to 8 doses.

An Ounce of Prevention

There's not much you can do to prevent this common infection, except the obvious: Keep your child away from a playmate who has come down with the disease.

When to Call for Help

The high fever that accompanies roseola can cause some children to have convulsions, also known as febrile seizure. Call for emergency assistance if your child has a seizure. After seeking help, watch your child closely: Do not try to restrain him during a convulsion, but listen for any changes in breathing. If he vomits during the seizure, turn his head to the side to minimize the risk of choking or inhaling vomit. Do your best to offer calming words of reassurance to comfort your child while you wait for help.

Runny Nose

They drool, they cry, and their little noses can run and run. Indeed, many children live up to the less-than-flattering phrase, "snotty-nosed kid." But all the dripping and running is Mother Nature's way of fighting viral infections and cleaning out bacteria and other irritants. The mucous membranes contain antibodies, which attack the viruses and wash them out of the body.

Runny noses, especially those that last longer than two weeks, can also be caused by allergies or hay fever. With allergic rhinitis the nasal secretions run clear and thin, rather than cloudy and thick as is common with colds. Hay fever often includes sneezing and watery eyes, as well (see page 58 for more information on allergies).

Runny noses can be annoying but they aren't usually serious. The constant drip can tickle the throat, causing a cough and sore throat. Or the mucus can clog the eustachian tubes in the ears and cause a painful ear infection. There are easy steps you can take at home to ease the irritation of a runny nose and reduce the risk of secondary infection.

Traditional Treatments

Blow, blow, blow. Buy your child his own package of tissue and teach him to blow his nose himself. If he needs a little incentive, offer a sticker as a prize each time he blows successfully. Teach him to toss used tissues in the trash right away to minimize the risk of passing a cold virus on to other children (or to you).

Lend a hand to those too young to blow. Infants and young toddlers won't be able to blow their noses on their own. Instead, you'll have to help them out by suctioning away the mucus with a bulb syringe (sold at most drugstores). Squeeze the bulb and insert the long tip into a nostril. As you release the bulb, the nasal secretions will be drawn into it. Your child may scream and yell when you do it, but he'll thank you (or wish that he could) after he calms down. Rinse out the bulb syringe and boil it for 10 minutes before using again, to discourage the spread of viruses and infection.

Wash up. After a sneeze, sniffle, or blow have your child wash his hands. Again, frequent hand-washing is the first line of defense against spreading the viruses that cause colds.

Check out the medicine cabinet. Depending on the cause of the sniffles, one of several drugs can help dry up the drip. Decongestants (such as those containing pseudoephedrine and ephedrine) shrink the mucous membranes and clear the nasal passages when a runny nose is caused by the common cold. Antihistamines can help when a runny nose is caused by an allergic reaction. Either drug should be used only when necessary, since they both have side effects: Decongestants can make some children nervous or ''wired,'' and antihistamines can cause drowsiness.

Rinse the nose. Saline (salt) drops can help wash the irritants out of your child's nose. Over-the-counter saline drops can be applied directly up your child's nose; for proper use, follow package directions.

Get the red out. A runny nose can result in a red nose and upper lip. To prevent irritation, rub a bit of petroleum jelly onto the affected area to keep it moist 2 or 3 times a day.

Natural Remedies

All of the natural remedies listed below can be used to supplement conventional medical treatment.

Diet and Nutrition

Use one or more of the remedies listed below. Dosage varies according to age; see the chart on pages 14–15 to determine to correct dose for your child. For good food sources of particular nutrients, see pages 9–13.

- Vitamin C helps reduce the inflammation that can be caused by a runny nose. Give your child 1 dose of vitamin C 3 times a day for 3 or 4 days.
- Zinc helps boost the immune system, which can dry up a runny nose. Give your child 1 dose of zinc a day for 3–4 days. (Excessive amounts of zinc can lead to nausea and vomiting, so don't exceed the dosage recommended on the package.)

Herbal

Use one or more of the remedies listed below. Dosage varies according to age; see the chart on page 25 to determine the correct dose for your child.

- Garlic helps fight bacterial infections and clear up a runny nose. Give your child 1 dose of odorless garlic twice daily (or open the capsule and dissolve its contents in a warm drink or soup).
- Thyme tea relieves sinus congestion and nasal pain. Give your child 1 dose of tea 2 or 3 times daily for as long as necessary.

Homeopathy

Use one homeopathic treatment at a time, based on your child's specific symptoms. For dosage information, see the chart on pages 31–37. Discontinue use if the symptoms disappear.

- *Hydrastis (Hydrastis canadensis)* 6c: Use if your child's nose is dripping all the time; the mucus is thin and drips down the back of throat. Give 4 times daily for up to 2 weeks.
- *Natrum mur. (Natrum muriaticum)* 6c: Use if the mucus looks like raw egg white, the nose is dry and sore, and your child experiences loss of smell and taste. Give 4 times daily for up to 2 weeks.
- *Sanguinaria (Sanguinaria canadensis)* 6c: Use if your child has profuse, yellow mucus and frequent sneezing. Give 4 times daily for up to 2 weeks.
- *Pulsatilla (Pulsatilla nigricans)* 6c: Use if your child has yellow or green mucus. Give 4 times daily for up to 2 weeks.

Acupressure

Use one or more of the acupressure points listed below. For a diagram showing the specific pressure points, see pages 40–41.

- Gates of Consciousness (Gallbladder 20): This point is located just below the base of the skull, in the hollow just outside the two large neck muscles.
- Welcoming Perfume (Large Intestine 20): Apply steady pressure on the point on either cheek, just outside each nostril.

An Ounce of Prevention

Runny noses are as common as the common cold. To prevent runny noses, keep your child away from other children with colds (which is easier said than done), and teach your child about the importance of regular hand-washing. If your child's nose starts dripping when he steps out in cold, windy air, wrap a scarf over his nose to warm the air before he inhales. For more information on runny noses caused by allergies, see the section on allergies on page 58.

When to Call for Help

Runny noses are nothing to run to the doctor about, unless there is evidence that an infection is present, in which case antibiotics may be needed to deal with the disease. Contact your pediatrician if the runny nose is accompanied by a high fever (103 degrees and above), if it lingers for more than 2 weeks, or if the mucus is yellow or green and has a strong odor. If you have an infant, call the doctor if the runny nose interferes with the baby's ability to eat and drink.

On rare occasions, a runny nose may be caused by a blocked nostril (after a toddler shoves a small object up the nose and doesn't tell you about it). In such cases, there may be a foul-smelling yellow or green discharge from one nostril. Contact your doctor to have the object removed.

Sore Throat

When your child has a sore throat, it hurts to swallow, eat, or even to drink a glass of water. Try to tolerate your child's crankiness; he will probably feel miserable for a couple of days.

Though both viruses and bacteria can cause sore throats, viruses are responsible for the majority of outbreaks. These viral infections clear up after a few days, and there's not much you can do to get rid of them (antibiotics won't work on viruses), though you can take steps to control the symptoms.

About 1 out of every 3 sore throats involves the streptococcal bacteria (or "strep throat"). Strep throat is most common in children over 3 years of age, and it involves a severe sore throat; red, swollen tonsils; and a temperature as high as 104 degrees. The common sore throat tends to start out with a scratchy feeling, then grow worse, but strep throat strikes suddenly—and severely.

Strep throat should be treated by a doctor. The doctor will prescribe antibiotics, to kill the bacteria and prevent possible complications, including kidney inflammation, throat abscesses, and rheumatic fever. Strep throat is relatively rare in adults, and is not the likely culprit if the sore throat is accompanied by symptoms of a common cold, such as runny nose and cough.

Traditional Treatments

Haven't got time for the pain. Acetaminophen can be used to control the pain and inflammation common to sore throats. Never administer aspirin (including "baby aspirin") to a child under age 18, since it can cause Reye's syndrome, a potentially fatal condition. For proper administration of acetaminophen, follow the package directions.

Keep it cool and wet. Your child's throat will feel better if it is kept moist. Offer your child cool water or flat ginger ale (the carbonation can irritate the throat and colas can be too acidic). Ice cream and popsicles provide both cool comfort and wet relief—and your child probably won't mind indulging in these tasty treats.

Humidify, humidify, humidify. Dry air can further irritate a tender throat, especially during the night. Running a humidifier or vaporizer in your child's bedroom will help to keep the air as moist as possible. Be sure to clean the appliance regularly, following the manufacturer's instructions on the proper method of doing so.

Natural Remedies

All of the natural remedies listed below can be used to supplement conventional medical treatment.

Diet and Nutrition
Use one or more of the remedies listed below. Dosage varies according to age; see the chart on pages 14–15 to determine to correct dose for your child. For good food sources of particular nutrients, see pages 9–13.

- Beta-carotene helps heal sore throats. Give your child 1 dose twice daily for 2 days.
- Vitamin C fights bacteria and helps reduce inflammation. Give your child 1 dose of vitamin C 3 times daily for 3 days.

Herbal
Use one or more of the remedies listed below. Dosage varies according to age; see the chart on page 25 to determine the correct dose for your child.

- An echinacea and goldenseal combination helps clear infection and boost the immune system. Give your child 1 dose

4 times daily for the first 2 days, then 1 dose three times daily for the next two or three days.

- Garlic helps kill bacteria while boosting the immune system. Give your child 1 dose of odorless garlic in capsule form once a day for 4 or 5 days, or follow package directions.

Homeopathy

Use one homeopathic treatment at a time, based on your child's specific symptoms. For dosage information, see the chart on pages 31–37. Discontinue use if the symptoms disappear.

- *Belladonna (Atropha belladonna)* 30x or 9c: Use if your child's tonsils, throat, and uvula are red and sore. Give 1 dose every hour for up to 3 doses.
- *Ferrum phos. (Ferrum phosphoricum)* 6x: Use if your child has a mild to moderate fever along with sore throat. Give 1 dose 3 times daily until fever breaks.
- *Phosphorus* 30x or 9c: Use if your child's sore throat is accompanied by hoarseness, and worsens in the evening. Give 1 dose 3 times daily for up to 2 days.
- *Phytolacca (Phytolacca decandra)* 12x or 6c: Use if your child has a dark, red throat and pain with swallowing that radiates back to the ears. Give 1 dose 4 times daily for up to 2 days.

Acupressure

Use one or more of the acupressure points listed below. For a diagram showing the specific pressure points, see pages 40–41.

- Heaven Rushing Out (Conception Vessel 22): This point is located at the base of the throat in the large hollow directly below the Adam's apple or voice box.
- Heavenly Pillar (Bladder 10): To find this point, place your fingers 1 child's finger width below the base of the skull on the muscles just outside the spine.
- Joining the Valley (Large Intestine 4): This is found at the highest spot of the muscle on the back of the hand that protrudes when the thumb and index finger are close together.

An Ounce of Prevention

Avoid exposing your child to airborne irritants such as cig-arette smoke, and try to keep your child away from friends and classmates suffering from colds or flu. You may also be able to minimize the frequency of a sore throat by dealing with a runny nose as soon as possible. (For more information on runny noses, see page 246.)

When to Call for Help

If you suspect your child's sore throat may actually involve strep, you should make a trip to the doctor to confirm your diagnosis and to start a course of antibiotics. Most run-of-the-mill sore throats are caused by viral infections that clear up on their own in a couple of days; a sore throat that lasts more than 3 days should also be checked by a doctor.

In addition, even with a viral infection you should call your doctor if your child experiences difficulty breathing or refuses to drink (which could cause dehydration).

Splinters

Splinters are an inevitable part of the rough-and-tumble world of childhood. When your child comes home with a palm full of splinters, take the tweezers in hand and get to work.

Traditional Treatments

- *Easier in than out.* If you can grab it, it's yours for the taking. Using a clean pair of tweezers or your fingernails, pull the splinter out, yanking it in the opposite direction from where it entered. Use a magnifying glass and plenty of light to make the job easier. If possible, sterilize the tweezers by putting them in boiling water for 2 or 3 minutes, by holding them over an open flame for 20–30 seconds, or by pouring an antiseptic such as rubbing alcohol over them.

- *Don't worry about it.* If you can't reach it, don't worry about leaving tiny splinter specks behind. Check on them after a day or 2. In most cases, your child's body will have naturally pushed them to the surface of the skin where they can be removed easily.
- *Soften 'em up.* Soak the area where the splinter is lodged in warm water for 10 or 15 minutes before trying to remove it. The water will soften the skin, and may force the splinter to the surface. If the splinter refuses to show itself, use a sterilized needle and gently scrape the skin around the splinter until you can reach it. Wash the area thoroughly with soap and water when you're finished. Go easy on the needlework; if the procedure requires too much poking and prodding, give up and call the doctor.

Natural Remedies

All of the natural remedies listed below can be used to supplement conventional medical treatment.

Herbal
Use one or more of the remedies listed below.

- After the splinter has been removed, apply calendula ointment to help prevent infection.
- If you can't grab the splinter with tweezers, try an herbal paste to draw it to the surface of the skin. Make a paste using slippery elm bark or fenugreek seeds (available at health food stores) and a bit of hot water. (Herbal companies also sell products already blended for just this purpose.) Smear the paste over the splintered area, then wrap it with gauze. Check every 4 hours and apply more paste, if necessary.

Homeopathy

For dosage information, see the chart on pages 31–37. Discontinue use if the symptoms disappear.

- *Silicea (Silicea terra)* 6c: Use if a splinter is embedded in the skin and cannot be reached with tweezers. To help the body push the splinter to the surface of the skin, give 1 dose 4 times daily for up to 3 days.

An Ounce of Prevention

Not every childhood mishap can be prevented; splinters fall into the unavoidable category, in most cases. Warn your child about possible splinters around wooden gyms and swing sets, as well as on piers and docks. At home, be sure that all wooden objects and railings are well-sanded and splinter-free, and, of course, keep wood scraps out of a child's reach in a workshop or garage.

When to Call for Help

If a splinter is deeply embedded in the skin or close to an eye, spare your child (and yourself) a lot of pain and suffering and have your doctor remove it. A medical professional will have sterile tools better suited for the job than most parents keep in the family first-aid kit.

After a splinter has been removed, a bit of redness can be expected, but bacteria can invade and cause infection. If the site is hot, swollen and oozes pus, contact your doctor; antibiotics may be needed.

Sprains and Strains

It goes with the turf: Few kids, especially active ones, can make it through childhood without suffering at least one sprain or muscle strain—whether it's caused by a stumble on the softball field, or a twisted ankle on the stairs, or a nasty fall while in-line skating.

Strains and sprains should be treated the same way. A strain involves overusing or overstretching a *muscle*, which causes tiny tears in the muscle tissue; sprains are caused by overusing or overstretching the *ligaments*, the tough bands of tissue that connect the bones.

Both strains and sprains cause pain, swelling, and black-and-blue marks in the affected areas. In many cases, it is difficult or impossible to determine whether the underlying bone has been fractured or broken, so most injuries serious enough to cause these symptoms should be checked by a medical professional.

Traditional Treatment

R—I—C—E is nice. Remember the acronym RICE: rest, ice, compression, and elevation. Rest the injury and avoid putting pressure on it. Wrap ice in a towel and apply it to the area for 30 minutes to reduce swelling. (A bag of frozen peas or a cold can of soda can work well if ice is not available.) If the area shows signs of swelling, apply the ice for 30 minutes, then remove it for 15 minutes, repeating the same procedure for the next few hours. After icing, wrap the injured area in an elastic bandage to provide support and to minimize swelling and bleeding. (Don't wrap the injury so tightly that you cut off circulation, though.) Finally, if possible, elevate the injured area above heart level to reduce swelling.

Take it easy. It takes time for an injury to heal. You should encourage your child to ease up on an injured limb for several weeks—it will take 4–6 weeks for the injured area to return to full strength. Trying to do too much too early can result in reinjury.

Natural Remedies

All of the natural remedies listed below can be used to supplement conventional medical treatment.

Diet and Nutrition

Use one or more of the remedies listed below. Dosage varies according to age; see the chart on pages 14–15 to determine to correct dose for your child. For good food sources of particular nutrients, see pages 9–13.

- Vitamin C with bioflavonoids helps repair and strengthen connective tissue, in addition to serving as an effective anti-inflammatory. Give your child 1 dose 3 times daily for 1 week.
- Zinc promotes tissue repair and helps the bones absorb calcium. Give your child 1 dose 3 times daily for 3 or 4 days.

Herbal

Use one or more of the remedies listed below.

- Arnica soothes muscles and reduces bruising after trauma or shock. Apply arnica externally using either an ointment or lotion. (Don't use on broken skin since it can cause irritation.)
- Comfrey is widely used as a "bone knitter" and healer; the herb promotes growth of new cells and reduces inflammation. Make a comfrey poultice by mixing 3 tablespoons of powdered herb with 3 ounces of hot water, then apply the paste directly to the injured area and cover with a clean cloth or bandage. Several hours later, remove the poultice and massage the area with comfrey-containing salves or ointments, available at health food stores.

Homeopathy

Use one homeopathic treatment at a time, based on your child's specific symptoms. For dosage information, see the chart on pages 31–37. Discontinue use if the symptoms disappear.

- *Arnica (Arnica montana)* 6c: If your child strains or sprains a muscle, try this remedy first. Give 1 dose every half hour for up to 10 doses.
- *Bryonia (Bryonia alba)* 6c: Use if the joint is very swollen and the slightest movement causes pain. Give 1 dose every ½ hour for up to 10 doses.
- *Rhus tox. (Rhus toxicodendron)* 6c: Use if the muscle hurts when your child starts to move, but the pain eases with continued movement. Give 1 dose every ½ hour for up to 10 doses.

Acupressure

For a diagram showing the specific pressure point, see pages 40–41.

- Wilderness Mound (Gallbladder 40): In the large hollow directly in front of the outer anklebone (for ankle sprains).

An Ounce of Prevention

If your child is an athlete, it is almost impossible to prevent all sprains and strains, but you can do your best to minimize his chances. Buy high-quality sports goods and equipment and make sure they fit your child properly. Make sure your local playing field is relatively free of potholes or rough spots that could cause your child to trip or twist an ankle.

Encourage your child to warm up and stretch before participating in a sporting event. Don't allow your child to join in any contact sport before he is physically and mentally mature enough to follow the rules and handle the roughhousing.

When to Call for Help

Muscle strains and sprains require medical attention to rule out the possibility of a fracture. Treat an injury as if it were a break, until you can rule out that possibility (usually by getting an X ray). If you don't suspect a fracture but the condition does not improve within 24 hours, contact your doctor.

Stomachache

Not many parents will make it to their child's high school graduation without at least one memory of their little one complaining, "My tummy hurts." Stomachaches are common childhood complaints, whether they are caused by gas, hunger, indigestion, constipation, food poisoning, food allergy, or emotional upset.

In some cases, the only symptom is an achy or crampy tummy; other times the stomachache is a prelude to nausea, vomiting, and sometimes diarrhea. Most stomachaches are nothing to worry about and will disappear within a half hour or so. Those that last more than a few hours are probably caused by food poisoning or infection. (See page 168 for more information on food poisoning.)

Traditional Treatments

Warm up the tummy. A heating pad (on the lowest setting) or a hot-water bottle can provide significant comfort to a child with tummy trouble. The warmth soothes and eases the stomach pain. (To avoid burns, don't allow your child to lie on top of the heating pad, and do not leave the child unattended.)

Skip the chow. When your child complains of a stomachache, serve clear liquids, such as chicken broth, flat ginger ale, and water. Introduce bland foods—bananas, rice, applesauce, and toast—when your child asks for something more filling.

Talk it over. If your child's stomachaches seem to follow the school calendar, showing up on Monday and clearing up by the weekend, talk to your child about possible pressures at school. Don't assume that your child is faking the illness; the symptoms can be real responses to anxieties facing him at school. Discuss the problem with your child, and contact a school guidance counselor or other professional if you feel you need additional help getting to the heart of the problem.

Need a bathroom break? Constipation can cause stomachache and/or an impacted bowel. For more information on constipation, see page 121.

Try a rub-down. Some stomachaches, especially those caused by gas or constipation, respond to gentle massage. Ask your child to lie down and relax. Gently massage his abdomen clockwise, following the pattern of the digestive system—starting below the rib cage, then circling around the top of the groin area and up to the belly. Repeat this soothing massage for several minutes, rubbing with massage oil if you and your child prefer.

Natural Remedies

All of the natural remedies listed below can be used to supplement conventional medical treatment.

Diet and Nutrition

Use one or more of the remedies listed below. Dosage varies according to age; see the chart on pages 14–15 to determine to correct dose for your child. Some vitamins can be used topically, as noted. For good food sources of particular nutrients, see pages 9–13.

- Lactobacillus acidophilus can help relieve and prevent stomachache and nausea by restoring beneficial bacteria to the intestines. Give your child 1 dose 3 times daily for 2 weeks, following dosage information on the product label. One

serving daily of yogurt with live cultures can also help restore intestinal bacteria.
* Provide your child with a balanced diet, including high-fiber, low-fat, and low-sugar foods.

Herbal
Use one or more of the remedies listed below. Dosage varies according to age; see the chart on page 25 to determine the correct dose for your child.

* Ginger tea can help ease stomachache and minimize nausea. Give your child 1 dose 2 or 3 times daily for up to 3 days. (If your child doesn't like the taste of the tea, dilute it with as much apple juice as necessary to make it palatable.)
* Licorice root can help relax and settle an achy stomach. Give your child 1 dose of licorice root tea 3 times daily for up to 3 days.

Homeopathy
Use one homeopathic treatment at a time, based on your child's specific symptoms. For dosage information, see the chart on pages 31–37 . Discontinue use if the symptoms disappear.

* *Aconite (Aconitum napellus)* 30c: Use if the stomachache is causing your child to feel frightened or panicky. Give 1 dose every 5 minutes for up to 6 doses.
* *Ignatia (Ignatia amara)* 30x or 9c: Use if your child's complaints appear to be linked to emotional stress. Give 1 dose 3 times daily for up to 3 days.
* *Nux (Strychnos nux vomica)* 30x or 9c: Use if your child develops a stomachache after overeating, or after having too much fried food. Give 1 dose 3 times daily for up to 6 doses.

Acupressure
Use one or more of the acupressure points listed below. For a diagram showing the specific pressure points, see pages 40–41.

* Abdominal Sorrow (Spleen 16): This point is located below the edge of the rib cage, ½ inch in from the nipple line.

- Inner Gate (Pericardium 6): To find this point, place your fingers in the middle of the inner side of the forearm 2½ child's finger widths from the wrist crease.
- Three Mile Point (Stomach 36): Apply steady pressure on the point 4 child's finger widths below the kneecap, 1 child's finger width to the outside of the shinbone. If you are on the correct spot, a muscle will flex as the foot is moved up and down.

An Ounce of Prevention

Stomachaches—both real and imagined—are part of childhood. As a parent, it's your job to decipher when complaints of a stomachache are nothing more than a ploy to avoid school on a test day, and when the complaint is the real thing. You can prevent some of the imaginary stomachaches by encouraging your child to talk about his feelings and stresses. You can prevent some of the real ones by teaching your child to wash his hands regularly and to avoid putting dirty fingers in his mouth. (Many bacterial and viral infections are spread by hand-to-mouth contact.)

Sometimes kids develop stomach pains by overeating or by gobbling their food too quickly. Encourage your child to take his time and stop eating when he feels satisfied.

When to Call for Help

Almost all stomachaches clear up without the need for a doctor visit. However, you should be on the lookout for signs of complications, including severe pain (especially on the right side of the abdomen) and high fever, which could indicate appendicitis. Also contact your doctor if your child develops projectile vomiting, blood in the vomit, or pain that lasts for more than 3 hours.

Stuffy Nose

Your heart has to go out to the wide-eyed kid who looks at you and pleads in a nasal voice, "Help, I can't breathe," wanting you to reach down and make it all better. If only it were that easy.

Stuffy noses usually stem from a cold virus or allergen that has settled in the nasal passages. As the virus or allergen irritates the membranes in the nose, the blood vessels swell and secrete mucus, until eventually the nasal passage is completely blocked. Inhale, nothing happens; exhale, nothing happens.

Stuffy noses can be kind of scary, especially to young children who don't understand what is happening to them and to babies who can't nurse without occasionally gasping for air. Take heart, the condition will soon pass, especially if you follow these tips designed to help clear the airways.

Traditional Treatments

Wetter is better. Moist warm air will help loosen the mucus and soothe the nasal passages. Try turning on a hot shower and sitting in the bathroom for 20 or 30 minutes with your child. Or run a vaporizer or humidifier in your child's bedroom at night to keep the air as humid as possible. (Make sure to clean the machine regularly, following the manufacturer's instructions.)

Wetter is better, part 2. If your child can't breathe through his nose, he's breathing through his mouth, which can be dehydrating and leave your child with a dry, sticky mouth. Drinking water and other clear fluids, such as flat ginger ale and clear broths, prevents dry mouth, helps fight dehydration, and keeps the mucus freely flowing.

Clear the way. Babies may need a little extra help clearing their nasal passages. Use a nasal aspirator or bulb syringe (available at any drugstore) to suction out the mucus. Squeeze the bulb end of a clean aspirator and gently insert it into your baby's nostril. Release the bulb and it will draw in the nasal mucus, clearing the secretions. Boil the aspirator for 10 minutes to sterilize it before storing it in your medicine cabinet.

Say 'yes' to nose drops. Saltwater nose drops, whether store-bought or homemade, help clear the nasal passages. To make your own, mix 1/4 teaspoon of salt with 1/2 cup of warm water. Administer 1 or 2 drops per nostril, wait a few minutes, then suction out the secretions using a nasal aspirator (older kids can just blow their nose). Remember, don't put the eyedropper back in the saline solution after putting it in your child's nose, or you'll contaminate the leftover solution. Sterilize by boiling both the dropper and the aspirator after you've finished.

Don't believe the advertising. Over-the-counter decongestants promise to ease your child's stuffy nose, but the fine print acknowledges that some children will become drowsy and others irritable and keyed up. You won't know how your child will react the drug, but consider the possible side effects before putting out a measuring spoon. And, of course, if you do decide to administer a decongestant, follow the label directions for the appropriate dose for your child.

Natural Remedies

All of the natural remedies listed below can be used to supplement conventional medical treatment.

Diet and Nutrition

Use one or more of the remedies listed below. Dosage varies according to age; see the chart on pages 14–15 to determine to correct dose for your child. For good food sources of particular nutrients, see pages 9–13.

- Beta-carotene helps heal the mucous membranes. Give your child 1 dose 3 times a day for 3 or 4 days.
- Vitamin C with bioflavonoids helps reduce inflammation and fight infection. Give your child 1 dose of each 3 times a day for 3 or 4 days.

Herbal

Use one or more of the remedies listed below. Dosage varies according to age; see the chart on page 25 to determine the correct dose for your child.

- Echinacea and goldenseal fight infection and boost the immune system. Give your child 1 dose of an echinacea and goldenseal combination formula every 2 hours for up to 3 doses.
- Garlic helps fight bacterial infections. If your child's stuffy nose is not caused by allergies, give your child 1 dose of odorless garlic once a day for 1 week.

Homeopathy

Use one homeopathic treatment at a time, based on your child's specific symptoms. For dosage information, see the chart on pages 31–37. Discontinue use if the symptoms disappear.

- *Belladonna (Atropha belladonna)* 30c: Use if your child's congestion comes on suddenly and the sinuses are affected. Give 1 dose every 2 hours for up to 2 days.
- *Kali bichrom. (Kali bichromicum)* 6c: Use if your child's nose is blocked on one side. Give 1 dose every 2 hours for up to 2 days.
- *Silicea (Silicea terra)* 6c: Use if your child experiences throbbing pain in the sinuses. Give 1 dose every 2 hours for up to 2 days.

Acupressure

Use one or more of the acupressure points listed below. For a diagram showing the specific pressure points, see pages 40–41.

- Drilling Bamboo (Bladder 2): This point is located in the indentations of the eye sockets, on either side of where the bridge of the nose meets the ridge of the eyebrows.
- Facial Beauty (Stomach 3): To find this point, place your fingers at the bottom of the cheekbones, directly below the pupils.
- Gates of Consciousness (Gallbladder 20): Apply steady pressure to the point on the base of the skull, just outside the hollow formed by the muscles in the center of the neck.
- Joining the Valley (Large Intestine 4): This point is located at the highest spot of the muscle on the back of the hand that protrudes when the thumb and index finger are closest together.

An Ounce of Prevention

Stuffy noses are part of growing up. But you can avoid some stuffy-nose episodes by practicing good hygiene (especially hand-washing) and by avoiding sick playmates. If the stuffiness stems from an allergic reaction, eliminate as many known or suspected allergens as you can. (See page 58 for more information on allergies.)

When to Call for Help

Call your pediatrician if your infant develops a stuffy nose that interferes with nursing or feeding. With older children, call the doctor if the stuffiness is accompanied by a fever of 103 degrees F or if it lasts more than 1 week without improvement.

Sunburn

With sunburn, your child will pay now and pay later: suffering a red and painful burn for several days after excessive sun exposure, and facing an increased risk of skin cancer later in life.

Sunburn is caused by prolonged exposure to radiation from the sun. Most sunburns involve first-degree burns (the outer layer of the skin becomes red and painful), but more intense exposure can result in second-degree burns (the skin blisters and swells). Severe sunburns can cause nausea, chills, and fever, as well as that painfully familiar stinging.

Don't be lulled into a false sense of security simply because your child is sitting under a beach umbrella or wearing a T-shirt. The sun's burning rays can be reflected off the water or sand, causing problems even for those sitting in the shade. While wearing a T-shirt provides some sun protection, most fabrics are woven loosely and allow the sun's rays to penetrate. The only ways to avoid sunburn are to avoid the sun or liberally apply sunscreen.

You shouldn't assume that you can prevent your child from developing a sunburn by keeping an eye on his skin as it changes color. What initially appears as a pinkish tint will continue to grow redder and more painful as the sunburn develops over the 6–48 hours after exposure. If, despite your efforts, your child winds up with a painful burn, the following remedies can provide relief.

Traditional Treatments

- *Take a cold shower.* Or, better yet, a cool bath. Hot water will sting, but cool water can comfort the burning, red-hot skin. Adding oatmeal or Aveeno treatment to the bathwater

267

can also help soothe the skin. If you can't give your child a bath immediately, try cool, wet compresses until you reach home.

- *Turn to the medicine cabinet.* Ease the pain with acetaminophen or ibuprofen. If the burn turns itchy after several days, try an over-the-counter antihistamine. Follow package directions for both products. Do not give a child under age 18 aspirin (including "baby aspirin"), due to the risk of developing Reye's syndrome, a potentially fatal condition.
- *Skip the sprays.* Anesthetic sprays, such as those containing benzocaine, can help stop the stinging burn, but they can also cause an allergic reaction in some children. You don't want to deal with a skin reaction on top of a sunburn, so avoid using these chemicals to dull the sting.

Natural Remedies

All of the natural remedies listed below can be used to supplement conventional medical treatment.

Diet and Nutrition
Dosage varies according to age; see the chart on pages 14–15 to determine to correct dose for your child. For good food sources of particular nutrients, see pages 9–13.

- Zinc boosts the immune system and aids healing. Give your child 1 dose of zinc once a day for 7 days after a sunburn.

Herbal
Use one or more of the remedies listed below. Dosage varies according to age; see the chart on page 25 to determine the correct dose for your child.

- Aloe vera soothes and cools sunburned skin. Rub the gel directly onto the injured skin as often as necessary.
- Comfrey root promotes healing and can help cool the skin. Make comfrey-root tea by adding 1 teaspoon of dried herb to 1 cup of boiling water and steeping for 10 minutes. Allow the tea to cool, then soak a clean washcloth in the tea

and apply the compress to the sunburned skin. *Comfrey should not be taken internally.*

Homeopathy
Use one homeopathic treatment at a time, based on your child's specific symptoms. For dosage information, see the chart on pages 31–37. Discontinue use if the symptoms disappear.

- *Sol* 30c: Use if your child develops a sunburn. Give 1 dose every 4 hours for up to 8 doses.
- *Ferrum phos. (Ferrum phosphoricum)* 12x or 6c: Use if your child develops a fever along with the sunburn. Give 1 dose right after the burn and another an hour later.

An Ounce of Prevention

You know better. Excessive sun exposure and sunburn contribute to skin cancer, including malignant melanoma. It's up to you to do all you can to stop your child from getting overdone in the sun:

- *Slather on the sunscreen.* Thoroughly apply sunscreen ½ hour before allowing your child to go outdoors. Reapply sunscreens—including waterproof products—every 3 or 4 hours throughout the day. Choose a sunscreen with an SPF (sun protection factor) of 15 or higher.
- *Stock up every year.* The active ingredients in sunscreens don't last from one season to the next. Buy a new bottle or tube every year.
- *Can you see your shadow?* Stay out of the sun as much as possible during the peak burning hours of 10 A.M. to 3 P.M. That rule applies even on cloudy, overcast days; about 80 percent of the sun's burning rays pass right through the clouds.
- *Wear a hat.* Get your child used to wearing a hat as a baby, and enforce the rule as he gets older. Choose a hat with a wide brim to protect the ears, an often overlooked spot when it comes to applying sunscreen.

When to Call for Help

Most first-degree sunburns can be treated at home, but blistering second-degree burns should be seen by a physician. Also, bring your child to the doctor if he complains of nausea, chills, or fever.

Teething

At first, you may not be sure what's wrong with your little one: He's fussy, he won't eat, and he drools all over everything. Then, that first spot of white erupts—and your baby's toothless grin becomes a thing of the past.

Most children sprout their first tooth when they're 6 months old. After that, on average, a new tooth shows up every month. Every child is different, but the first teeth to break through are usually the two middle teeth on the bottom; the molars are the last to break through. Your child's smile will change month by month until the full set of 20 baby (primary) teeth is in at about age 2½. The complete set includes 8 incisors for cutting, 4 canines for tearing, and 8 molars for crushing.

The permanent teeth usually begin coming in at age 6 or 7. The baby tooth is loosened as the permanent tooth begins to emerge. Permanent teeth usually do not cause the same pain as baby teeth, except for the final molars (wisdom teeth), which generally appear in the late teens or early twenties.

Traditional Treatments

Let him chew it over. The pressure of chewing or rubbing the gums can provide considerable relief to a teething infant. Wash your hands, then rub your baby's gums with your finger, or give him a clean, cold, wet washcloth to chew on. If your baby has moved on to some solid foods, consider providing a cold carrot stick or a frozen bagel to chomp on. Of course, a teething ring will also do the trick. (Do not freeze teething rings, since they can cause frostbite if held directly against the skin for an extended period of time.)

Treat the pain. Teething pain may not be caused by illness or trauma, but the pain deserves to be treated nonetheless. Consider using an over-the-counter pain reliever, particularly if the pain interferes with a good night's sleep (for your baby or for you). Remember, a child should never be given aspirin (including "baby aspirin"), which can cause Reye's syndrome, a potentially fatal condition.

Numb the gums. If you've tried everything and nothing seems to work, try an over-the-counter gum preparation. Follow the directions on the package for appropriate usage.

Natural Remedies

All of the natural remedies listed below can be used to supplement conventional medical treatment.

Herbal
Use one or more of the remedies listed below.

- Both clove oil and tea tree oil are soothing to the gums. Mix 1 drop of either oil to 5 drops of olive oil and massage the mixture into your baby's gums. If your baby wants to bite anything put in his mouth, mix 10–15 drops of either oil with a ½ cup of water, saturate a clean cloth with the mixture and apply to the gums.

Homeopathy
Use one homeopathic treatment at a time, based on your child's specific symptoms. For dosage information, see the chart on pages 31–37. Discontinue use if the symptoms disappear.

- *Aconite (Aconitum napellus)* 30c: Use if your child develops acute pain and a fever. Give 1 dose every ½ hour for up to 10 doses.

- *Actaea (Actaea spicata)* 6c: Use if your child seems nervous and restless. Give 1 dose every ½ hour for up to 10 doses.
- *Chamomilla (Chamomilla vulgaris)* 30c: Use if your child is irritable with hot, red cheeks. Give 1 dose every ½ hour for up to 10 doses.

Acupressure

Use one or more of the acupressure points listed below. For a diagram showing the specific pressure points, see pages 40–41.

- Listening Place (Small Intestine 19): This point is located directly in front of the ear opening in a depression that deepens when the mouth is open.
- Facial Beauty (Stomach 3): To find this point, place your fingers at the bottom of the cheekbones, below the pupil of the eye.
- Joining the Valley (Large Intestine 4): Apply steady pressure in the webbing between the thumb and index finger, at the highest spot of the muscle that protrudes when the thumb and index finger are brought closest together.
- Wind Screen (Triple Warmer 17): This point is located in the indentation behind the earlobe.

An Ounce of Prevention

You can't stop your baby from growing up, and you can't stop those first teeth from breaking through your baby's smooth, pink gums. All you can do is take steps to ease the pain—and provide as much comfort as possible.

When to Call for Help

Teething may make your child (and you) miserable for a few days, but it should not cause any serious medical complications. Though unpleasant, chewing, drooling, crying, and rubbing swollen gums are all perfectly normal. Fever, vomiting, and diarrhea sometimes accompany teething, but these symptoms result from colds and other illnesses, not the teething process itself. If your baby experiences cold or flu symptoms, treat them accordingly, or contact your pediatrician.

Tick Bites and Lyme Disease

They're out there, waiting. Every summer, ticks feast on unsuspecting child-sized hosts—and their parents. While these tiny arachnids have always been a seasonal annoyance, these days they can also be responsible for spreading Lyme disease, a condition characterized by flu-like symptoms, a bull's-eye rash, joint inflammation, and chronic arthritis. Though less common, ticks have been implicated in spreading other diseases as well, including Rocky Mountain Spotted Fever, Colorado Tick Fever, and Ehrlichiosis.

Quite simply, ticks attach themselves to their hosts and suck their blood. Unfortunately, they drink slowly, so bacteria have plenty of time to enter and exit as the tick enjoys its meal. While most tick bites leave their hosts with a few drops less blood, they don't cause much harm. However, some ticks can spread a number of diseases, including Lyme disease, which is caused by the bacterium *borrelia burgdorferi*. The vast majority of cases of Lyme disease occur in the Northeast; however, the disease has reached virtually every state, so all parents should keep an eye out for signs of the illness.

Traditional Treatments

- *Check every square inch.* When your child comes in from playing outside in a woody area, perform a detailed tick check. Follow this full body check with a shower and shampoo to wash off any ticks you might not have spotted. (In the early spring, deer ticks can be the size of a pinhead.)

- *Leave my kid alone.* A crawling tick can be scooped up and flushed down the toilet, but a tick that has buried its head must be carefully removed. If possible, use tweezers; some bacteria may be spread through your (unbroken) skin if you grab the tick with your fingers. Place the tweezers as close to the skin as possible, then squeeze and pull straight away, without twisting. (You don't want to leave the mouth parts behind because they can become infected.)

- *What not to do.* Don't listen to advice from people who tell you to burn the tick with a cigarette butt or smother it with nail polish. You risk burning the child with the cigarette; the nail-polish technique takes too long—it could take hours to suffocate a tick, and it will be pumping your child full of infectious bacteria the entire time.

- *Clean it up.* After the tick has been removed, thoroughly clean the area with soap and water, then apply an antiseptic ointment.

- *Look for the bull's-eye.* Once your child is tick-free, begin watching for signs of Lyme disease. A distinctive oval bull's-eye rash often appears in the early stages of the disease. At the same time, most people with Lyme disease complain of fever, headache, lethargy, muscle pain, nausea, and vomiting. The final stage of the disease can include joint pain and arthritis-like symptoms, which sometimes don't show up for as long as 2 years after the initial infection. Once it is detected, Lyme disease *can* be treated, usually with antibiotics.

Natural Remedies

All of the natural remedies listed below can be used to supplement conventional medical treatment.

Diet and Nutrition

Use one or more of the remedies listed below. Dosage varies according to age; see the chart on pages 14–15 to determine to correct dose for your child. For good food sources of particular nutrients, see pages 9–13.

- Vitamin C fights bacteria and reduces inflammation. Give your child 1 dose of vitamin C twice a day for 1–2 weeks after a tick bite.
- Zinc promotes healing and stimulates the immune system. Give your child 1 dose of zinc twice a day for 5–7 days.

Herbal
Use one or more of the remedies listed below.

- After removing a tick, apply calendula ointment to ease the pain and lower the risk of infection. Apply directly to the site twice daily for 1 or 2 days.
- Tea tree oil is an antiseptic that can reduce the risk of infection at the wound site. Apply directly to the site twice daily for 1 or 2 days.

An Ounce of Prevention

When your child heads out to play in a wooded or grassy area where ticks may be lurking, dress him in long pants and a long-sleeved shirt. Long socks and a hat will also help. The less flesh showing, the better. Stick to light-colored clothes, which will make the ticks easier to spot.

When your child comes home, give him a careful once over from head to toe, especially around the hairline and in tight spots like waistbands. Remove any ticks as soon as possible; it usually takes 24 hours for an implanted tick to spread disease (unless it is disrupted when you try to remove it).

If you have a family pet, talk to your veterinarian about tick repellents and give the animal regulars tick-checks so that you can spot ticks before they fall off inside your home and lay eggs.

When to Call for Help

Lyme disease responds best to early diagnosis and treatment. If you notice a bull's-eye rash or any other suspicious rash, call your doctor. In addition, if your child complains of stiff joints or excessive achiness, consider having the doctor test for Lyme disease.

Tooth Broken or Knocked Out

A toothless grin looks endearing on a newborn, but not nearly so appealing on an older child who has lost or damaged a tooth in a sporting injury or other accident. Still, hundreds of thousands of kids get their teeth knocked out each year.

If your child suffers a blow strong enough to crack, break, or knock out a tooth, you should visit the dentist to determine the extent of the damage. Loss of a baby tooth may not require any special treatment, but the dentist might want to use a bridge or "spacer" to prevent the other teeth from shifting out of place.

Damage to a permanent tooth demands prompt attention, since you don't get second chances with permanent teeth. Quick thinking and even quicker action will increase the odds that the tooth can be successfully reimplanted or repaired.

Traditional Treatments

• *Assessing the Damage.* Check your child's mouth carefully. If a tooth looks cracked but is not bleeding, then the interior of the tooth, known as the pulp, has not been ruptured. Chances are good you'd know if your child has a deeply fractured tooth; a crack that reaches the pulp causes excruciating pain. In most cases, your dentist can repair a simple crack.

- *Hanging by a thread.* A tooth that has been loosened but remains attached to the socket by the ligament should be left in place. Have your child gently bite down to hold it in place, and get him to the dentist for an emergency visit.
- *It's a knock-out.* First things first: Find the missing tooth. Hold it by the crown, taking special care not to touch the root or ligament that once held the tooth to the socket. Your goal is to get the tooth cleaned and back in the child's mouth as soon as possible.
- *The sooner the better.* Don't try to clean off the tooth by scraping it; if you pull the ligament off the tooth, it cannot be reattached to the socket. Time is of the essence: If the tooth and ligament are treated and put in place in the mouth within 15–30 minutes, the tooth can be successfully re-planted about 90 percent of the time. Work as quickly as possible, but don't watch the clock. Do everything you can to locate and replace the tooth, even if it takes longer. In some cases, your efforts will be rewarded and the tooth will be spared.
- *Keep it wet.* You need to keep the tooth and the ligament from drying out on the trip to the dentist. Rinse the tooth in saline contact lens solution or milk, then put it back in the socket if your child is old enough not to swallow it. Have your child bite down on a clean rag or cloth to hold it in place until you reach the dentist. Putting the tooth in the socket may also prevent the socket from clotting over. WARNING: Don't rinse the tooth in tap water because in most areas it contains chlorine, which can damage the ligament.
- *There's no place like home.* But if your child can't keep the tooth in its socket during the ride to the dentist's office, then submerge it in a glass of milk, which has the right pH to protect the ligament. As a last resort, put the tooth in your own mouth to keep it moist and protected.

Natural Remedies

All of the natural remedies listed below can be used to supplement conventional medical treatment.

Diet and Nutrition

- Banish carbonated beverages from your child's diet. The highly acidic sodas can damage calcium in tooth enamel, and also slow recovery time for a broken tooth.

Herbal

- Apply a moistened black or green tea bag to the site of the injury if it is bleeding. The tannins in the tea constrict blood vessels and slow bleeding.

Homeopathy

For dosage information, see the chart on pages 31–37. Discontinue use if the symptoms disappear.

- *Arnica (Arnica montana)* 12x: Use after trauma to the mouth. Give 1 dose every 4 hours, for up to 3 doses.

Acupressure

Use one or more of the acupressure points listed below. For a diagram showing the specific pressure points, see pages 40–41.

- Facial Beauty (Stomach 3): This point is located at the bottom of the cheekbone, below the pupil of the eye.
- Joining the Valley (Large Intestine 4): To find this point, place your fingers in the webbing between the thumb and index finger, at the highest spot of the muscle that protrudes when the thumb and index finger are brought closest together.
- Listening Place (Small Intestine 19): Apply steady pressure to the point directly in front of the ear opening in the depression that deepens when the mouth opens.
- Wind Screen (Triple Warmer 17): This point is located in the indentation behind the earlobe.

An Ounce of Prevention

If your child participates in hazardous sporting activities, make sure he wears a protective mouth guard, which is available at sporting good stores. You can't always prevent dental disasters, but you can be prepared to think clearly and act swiftly if your child does damage a tooth.

When to Call for Help

Any dental mishap that involves a tooth that's cracked, broken, or knocked out demands immediate attention from a dentist. If your regular family dentist isn't available, head straight for the hospital emergency room.

Tooth Decay and Toothache

For most parents, it's a never-ending battle: You implore, cajole, and harass your child to brush his teeth, and your child responds by doing everything possible to avoid participating in this painless oral hygiene ritual. Tooth-brushing and flossing are the best ways to prevent cavities and keep teeth healthy. Neglected teeth grow progressively worse, sometimes resulting in toothache and serious dental problems.

Tooth decay occurs when bacterial plaque forms on the surface of the teeth. Though the layer of enamel covering the teeth is the hardest substance in the human body, it can be destroyed by the powerful acids created by oral bacteria. Over time, these acids eat away at the enamel, causing tooth decay. Left unattended, the decay will eventually expose the nerves in the tooth and cause excruciating tooth pain.

A toothache can indicate a number of problems, from something as harmless as a permanent tooth trying to edge out the baby tooth in its place, to a deep cavity or serious crack in the tooth enamel. The only way to be sure what's causing the pain is to take your child to the dentist. In the meantime, these strategies may help you make it through the night.

Traditional Treatments

Like taking candy from a baby. Don't let your baby go to sleep with a bottle of milk or juice in his mouth. The sugar in the drinks will form plaque behind the teeth, resulting in tooth decay. The problem of tooth decay in a baby's front teeth is so pervasive it has a name—"baby bottle syndrome."

Brush early, brush often. Before your child's first tooth breaks through, you can begin a ritual of wiping the gums with a clean, moist cloth after eating. This will prepare your child for tooth-brushing, when the time comes. As soon as your child has teeth, begin brushing with a soft-bristle baby toothbrush, without toothpaste at first. (Start using toothpaste when your child is about a year and a half.) You'll have to do most of the brushing until your child is much older. A rule of thumb: About the time your child is old enough to tie his own shoes, he should be ready to handle the responsibility of brushing on his own (with supervision, of course).

Make brushing fun. Turn tooth-brushing into a game. Let your child pick out an exciting toothbrush and a kid-flavored fluoride toothpaste. (A pea-sized dab of toothpaste is all your child needs.) Set a clock and have him brush for three minutes twice a day. For younger children, offer stickers or other minor rewards as incentives for a brushing job well done. Try using a dental irrigator or mechanical toothbrush—anything to keep your child interested and excited about oral hygiene.

Floss early, floss often. By the time your child is 3, he will probably have two back molars—it's time then for flossing. You'll have to handle this responsibility until your child is 8 or 9, since flossing takes a fair amount of coordination.

Pick the right dentist. Lots of people—both children and adults—don't like going to the dentist. Choosing a child-friendly dentist can go a long way toward alleviating your child's fear and making dental visits a little less scary. A good dentist will talk to your child and explain what is happening every step of the way. The more frequently you go to the dentist, the less likely serious (and painful) problems will arise, and the more likely the visits can continue to be positive and relatively painless.

Rinse away the pain. If your child has a toothache, offer a warm water rinse. The warmth and moisture may soothe the pain. In other cases, cold water may provide more relief; listen to what your child tells you.

Ice it down. If your child has a toothache, wrap ice in a clean towel and hold it against the jaw. The ice can soothe the pain and reduce swelling.

Do something for the pain. Open the medicine cabinet and try an over-the-counter painkiller such as acetaminophen to handle the tough pain. Follow package directions for correct dosage. Never give a child under age 18 aspirin (or ''baby aspirin''), because it can cause Reye's syndrome, a potentially fatal disorder.

Natural Remedies

All of the natural remedies listed below can be used to supplement conventional medical treatment.

Herbal
Use one or more of the remedies listed below.

- Clove oil is an oral anesthetic. If your child experiences a toothache, apply a drop or 2 of clove oil directly to the affected area for temporary relief.
- Fluoride helps protect the teeth and fight cavities. Fluoride is present in both black and green tea. If your tap water comes from a well or your municipal water supply does not fluoridate the water, give your child 1 cup of black or green tea daily to reduce the risk of cavities.

Homeopathy

Use one homeopathic treatment at a time, based on your child's specific symptoms. For dosage information, see the chart on pages 31–37. Discontinue use if the symptoms disappear.

- *Calcarea (Calcarea carbonia)* 6c: Use if your child has a problem with tooth decay and craves sweets. Give 1 dose twice daily for 3 weeks.
- *Coffea (Coffea cruda)* 6c: Use if your child has a toothache that is made worse by heat. Give 1 dose every 5 minutes for up to 10 doses.
- *Plantago (Plantago major)* 6c: Use if your child's tooth is ultra-sensitive, especially to cold air and pressure. Give 1 dose every 5 minutes for up to 10 doses.
- *Silicea (Silicea terra)* 6c: Use if your child has several decaying teeth. Give 1 dose twice daily for 3 weeks.

Acupressure

Use one or more of the acupressure points listed below. For a diagram showing the specific pressure points, see pages 40–41.

- Facial Beauty (Stomach 3): This point is located at the bottom of the cheekbone, below the pupil of the eye.
- Joining the Valley (Large Intestine 4): To find this point, place your fingers in the webbing between the thumb and index finger, at the highest spot of the muscle that protrudes when the thumb and index finger are brought closest together.
- Listening Place (Small Intestine 19): Apply steady pressure to the point directly in front of the ear opening in the depression that deepens when the mouth opens.
- Wind Screen (Triple Warmer 17): This point is located in the indentation behind the earlobe.

An Ounce of Prevention

With regular brushing, flossing, and dental checkups every 6 months after age 2, most kids can get through childhood with few, if any, cavities or toothaches. You can also reduce the likelihood of dental problems by following a few simple tips:

- Discourage between-meal snacking, unless your child brushes thoroughly after eating. Choose snacks wisely: Raw vegetables and cheese are much better for the teeth than cookies, chips, and dried fruit—sticky foods that get packed down around the molars. If your child can't brush because he is away from home and the necessary facilities aren't available, suggest that he rinse his mouth vigorously with plain water.
- Say no to soda and fruit juice, which are sugary and acidic, unless your child will brush up afterward. If you do allow sweet drinks, encourage your child to drink through a straw, which draws the beverage past the teeth, minimizing exposure to the sugars.
- Pass out the sugarless gum. Chewing sugarless gum for 15 or 20 minutes after eating can help clean the teeth. The gum pushes the trapped food away from the surface of the teeth, in addition to increasing the flow of saliva to the mouth, which helps wash away food particles and bacteria.

When to Call for Help

Don't wait for a dental emergency to contact the dentist; you should take your child in for a checkup and professional cleaning twice a year after age 2. If your child develops a toothache between appointments, call the dentist promptly. Toothaches, especially when accompanied by fever, can indicate an abscess.

Urinary Tract Infection

Urinary tract infections can make even the most loving child miserable. There are three common types of urinary tract infection: *urethritis* (infection of the tube that leads from the bladder to the outside of the body), *cystitis* (infection of the bladder), and *pyelitis* (infection of the kidneys). The urinary system is interconnected so infection tends to spread. The condition should be treated at the first sign of problems.

Urinary tract infections in infants usually stem from anatomical problems in the urinary tract, and should be dealt with by a physician immediately. In an infant, symptoms include: bloody urine, fever, vomiting, diarrhea, and irritability. Infections in older children usually result from bacterial contamination of the urinary tract, particularly from bacteria such as *E. coli*, which live in the bowel.

Some children have urinary tract infections without knowing it, but most episodes include a variety of symptoms, including frequent and painful urination, fever, back pain, redness of the genitals, minor incontinence, or cloudy urine. Untreated, the infection may either disappear on its own or spread to other parts of the urinary tract, so all infections should be treated as soon as possible.

Traditional Treatment

Drink up. Drink, drink, drink. Encourage your child to drink plenty of water. (Skip the soft drinks; many are acidic and can contribute to burning on urination.) The fluids help to flush the system and dilute the bacteria. When urine is left in the bladder, the bacteria have a chance to multiply. For example, the E. coli bacteria double in number every 20 minutes in the bladder. The bacteria cause the pain, so the more diluted the urine and the more often your child urinates, the less pain there should be.

Natural Remedies

All of the natural remedies listed below can be used to supplement conventional medical treatment.

Diet and Nutrition
Use one or more of the remedies listed below. Dosage varies according to age; see the chart on pages 14–15 to determine to correct dose for your child. For good food sources of particular nutrients, see pages 9–13.

- Cranberries really do help prevent and treat urinary tract infections. The berries contain a bacteria-fighting chemical known as hippuric acid. Give your child at least 3 8-ounce glasses of cranberry juice a day for as long as necessary.
- Lactobacillus acidophilus helps fight infection and encourages the growth of beneficial bacteria in the digestive and urinary tracts. Follow dosage information on the product label.

Herbal
Use one or more of the remedies listed below. Dosage varies according to age; see the chart on page 25 to determine the correct dose for your child.

- Garlic is a natural antibiotic. Give your child 1–3 doses of odorless garlic daily, until symptoms subside.
- Uva ursi is an antiseptic herb that can be effective against urinary tract infection. If your child is 6 or older, give 1 dose 3 times a day for 3–4 days. This herb can turn the urine dark green.

Homeopathy
For dosage information, see the chart on pages 31–37. Discontinue use if the symptoms disappear.

- *Cantharis (Cantharis lytta vesicatoria)* 12x or 6c: Use if your child experiences a burning sensation during urination. Give 1 dose 3–4 times daily for 3 days.

Acupressure

For a diagram showing the specific pressure point, see pages 40–41.

- Bigger Stream (Kidney 3): This point is located in the hollow midway between the protrusion of the inside anklebone and the Achilles tendon, which joins the back of the calf to the back of the heel.

An Ounce of Prevention

To prevent urinary tract infections, girls should be taught to wipe from front to back after bowel movements to avoid fecal contamination of the urethra. (Infants should always be wiped front to back during diaper changes for the same reason.) In addition, girls should use white, unscented toilet paper and mild soaps when bathing. Urinary tract infections are rare in boys. If your child develops symptoms, consult you doctor, since an anatomical problem may be involved.

When to Call for Help

Urinary tract infections should be taken seriously, especially in infants. Contact your doctor immediately if you suspect that your infant has a urinary tract infection. In addition, seek medical help if your child experiences fever, nausea or vomiting, pain in the lower back, or blood in the urine. These symptoms may indicate that the infection has spread to the kidneys.

Vomiting

Sometimes you can see it coming, other times it catches you by surprise, but there's no mistaking that telltale gagging sound and the mess that follows. Most bouts of vomiting don't last long. Whether caused by too much pepperoni pizza, an extra turn on the roller coaster, an emotional upset, a cold or flu virus, or a battle with gastroenteritis (a virus of the gastro-intestinal tract), most episodes of vomiting end when whatever is bothering the stomach makes its way out of your child's system.

With most cases of vomiting, the immediate risk is dehydration. Vomiting that lasts more than a day can lead to the loss of excessive amounts of fluid, especially if your child also experiences diarrhea. Still, most vomiting ends within 24 hours and leaves your child a bit worn out, but not seriously compromised.

Traditional Treatments

Settle down. When your child feels nauseated, allow him to skip meals and allow his stomach to calm down. If your child vomits for more than 2 or 3 hours, you should encourage him to consume over-the-counter oral rehydration fluids, which contain water, sugar, salt, and several other nutrients. Follow package directions for dosage information. Also offer ice chips or even a wet washcloth to suck on.

Don't start with an eight-course dinner. Ease back into the eating routine slowly. When your child asks for food, start by offering clear liquids and gelatin. If that stays down, move on to dry toast, crackers, rice, or potatoes. Lukewarm and flat

Coke or Pepsi—or better yet, the syrup alone—can also help settle the stomach.

Do not overfill. Overfeeding an infant can lead to spitting up or all-out vomiting. To minimize the problem, don't feed your baby more than he seems to want, and handle him gently during feeding and burping.

Natural Remedies

All of the natural remedies listed below can be used to supplement conventional medical treatment.

Diet and Nutrition

- Lactobacillus acidophilus helps ease nausea and vomiting by promoting the growth of healthy bacteria in the intestines. Give your child 1 dose 3 times daily for 1 week after the vomiting episode; see package label for dosage information.

Herbal

Use one or more of the remedies listed below. Dosage varies according to age; see the chart on page 25 to determine the correct dose for your child.

- Ginger tea helps relieve nausea and vomiting. Give your child 1 dose, up to 3 times daily, for 3 days. (If your child can't stomach the strong ginger taste, mix the tea with apple juice to sweeten it.)
- Licorice root tea soothes an unsettled stomach. Give your child 1 dose up to 3 times daily for 3 days. (Skip this remedy if your child has high blood pressure.)
- Peppermint tea can help calm a queasy tummy, especially if vomiting follows a heavy meal. Give your child 1 dose 2 or 3 times daily, for up to 3 days.

Homeopathy

Use one homeopathic treatment at a time, based on your child's specific symptoms. For dosage information, see the chart on pages 31–37. Discontinue use if the symptoms disappear.

- *Arsenicum (Arsenicum album)* 6c: Use if vomiting is accompanied by diarrhea. Give 1 dose every 15 minutes for up to 10 doses.
- *Ipecac (Cephaelis ipecacuanha)* 6c: Use if your child experiences persistent nausea and sharp abdominal pain. Give 1 dose every 15 minutes for up to 10 doses.
- *Pulsatilla (Pulsatilla nigricans)* 6c: Use if your child vomits after eating fatty food. Give 1 dose every 15 minutes for up to 10 doses.

Acupressure

Use one or more of the acupressure points listed below. For a diagram showing the specific pressure points, see pages 40–41.

- Grandfather Grandson (Spleen 4): This point is located on the bottom of the foot, 1 child's thumb width in back of the middle of the ball of the foot.
- Inner Gate (Pericardium 6): To find this point, place your fingers in the middle of the inner side of the forearm 2½ child's finger widths from the wrist crease.
- Three Mile Point (Stomach 36): Apply steady pressure on the point 4 child's finger widths below the kneecap, 1 finger width on the outside of the shinbone. If you are on the correct spot, a muscle will flex as the foot moves up and down.
- Travel Between (Liver 2): This point is located at the juncture of the big and second toes.

An Ounce of Prevention

To decrease the likelihood of your child picking up a "bug" (a virus or bacteria), teach him good hygiene, including regular hand-washing, especially before eating. In addition, try to make mealtimes as relaxed and comfortable as possible; discourage eating quickly and overeating, both of which can lead to nausea and vomiting.

When to Call for Help

Vomiting is an unpleasant—but an inevitable—part of childhood. Most episodes of vomiting are not serious, but you need to be on the lookout for signs of dehydration, including lack of urination (or very dark yellow urine), crying without tears, dry mucous membranes, listlessness, and drowsiness. If you can pinch your child's skin and it doesn't bounce back right away, he may be dehydrated.

Call the doctor if your child's vomiting lasts unabated for more than 24 hours. Also, call for help if your child experiences fever along with vomiting; if his stomach is bloated; if vomiting follows a head or stomach injury; if the vomit looks like coffee grounds; or if your infant has forceful, projectile vomiting. Each of these symptoms can indicate a more serious problem and warrant prompt medical attention.

Warts

They arrive unannounced and uninvited. All of a sudden you look down at your child's finger or elbow and there is a ghastly growth, a wart. Though unsightly, warts (also known as *verruca*) are nothing more than harmless little growths caused by viruses, known collectively as human papillomavirus, or HPV. They can appear at any age, but they are common among children since they suffer many minor cuts and scrapes, which allow the virus to enter the body. (That's also why they're common on the hands, fingers, elbows, and knees.)

Warts on the soles of the feet (called plantar warts) are

usually the only painful type of wart, though any growth will hurt if your child picks at it. Even if this type of wart does not cause outright pain, you may want to remove it to prevent its spread to other family members or other parts of the body. Given the chance, the virus will spread to a nearby area through an opening in the skin. Most common warts do not spread from person to person, but plantar warts are much more contagious.

Most childhood warts disappear within 2 years—but that can seem like a lifetime to a child who must endure taunting from playmates. The following remedies can help you rid your child of unwelcome warts, probably within a couple of weeks.

Traditional Treatments

Time heals. Warts have a limited lifespan, and they will eventually die off and disappear, though it could take months or years. If a wart isn't bothering your child, don't bother removing it, unless it spreads or your child is picking at it, which can encourage it to spread.

Make a wish. "I wish my wart would disappear." For some reason that scientists don't fully understand, some people are able to wish their warts away. Older kids may be able to visualize the growths melting or peeling away; younger kids may simply wish on a star. For 3–5 minutes a day, work with your child to think about the wart going away. It can't hurt to give it a try.

Go to the drugstore. If the magic of wishing doesn't work, the magic of over-the-counter medications just might. Most drugstores carry a number of nonprescription wart-removal products; follow the package instructions. (Most products contain salicylic acid either as a liquid, which is dripped onto the wart, or as a pad, which is cut to fit over the wart itself.) Since most products involve using a mild acid to burn the wart, don't use any product on a child who is under 6 years of age, since he may not be able to resist the temptation to pick at the affected area. The wart is gone when the fingerprint or normal skin ridges reappear.

Natural Remedies

All of the natural remedies listed below can be used to supplement conventional medical treatment.

Diet and Nutrition
Use one or more of the remedies listed below. Some vitamins can be used topically, as noted.

- Apply vitamin E directly to the wart and cover it with a bandage. Repeat this twice a day. (Be patient: This treatment can take weeks, or even months to work.)
- Vitamin C can kill the wart virus due to its high acidity. Crush vitamin C tablets and mix the powder with a few drops of water to form a paste. Apply the paste directly to the wart and cover with a bandage. The mixture will irritate the skin, then the wart will fall off over the course of several weeks.

Herbal
Use one or more of the remedies listed below.

- Banana peel contains a chemical that can kill the wart virus. Place a small amount of banana peel against the wart, and cover it with a bandage. Change the peel twice daily. Repeat for 2 weeks, or until the wart disappears.
- Place a crushed clove of garlic directly on the wart and cover it with a bandage. Blisters will form within 24 hours as the oil burns the skin. The wart should fall off within 1 week.

Homeopathy
Use one homeopathic treatment at a time, based on your child's specific symptoms. For dosage information, see the chart on pages 31–37. Discontinue use if the symptoms disappear.

- *Kali mur. (Kali muriaticum)* 6c: Use if your child develops warts on the hands. Give 1 dose twice daily for up to 3 weeks.
- *Natrum carb. (Natrum carbonicum)* 6c: Use if your child

develops warts on the toes. Give 1 dose twice daily for up to 3 weeks.
- *Sulphur* 6c: Use if your child develops warts that throb or burn. Give 1 dose twice daily for up to 3 weeks.

An Ounce of Prevention

Treat warts with respect. They are contagious and can spread to other parts of the body if they are irritated or picked. The virus can also spread from the hands to the face and mouth, so try to prevent your child from biting his fingernails or repeatedly touching his face.

The spread of plantar warts can be minimized by encouraging your child to wear pool slippers or flip-flops in the locker room and shower at school. If someone in your family has a plantar wart, encourage other family members to either use another bathroom, wear footwear in the bathroom, or disinfect the shower before hopping in. Take special care to kill this and other viruses by cleaning with disinfectants or chlorine bleach, after each use.

When to Call for Help

Warts come and go, usually with little fanfare. However, if your child is visiting the pediatrician's office, mention the wart and have your doctor look at it before you take steps to remove it. If you're not sure whether a growth is a wart or not, ask your doctor. Also, don't try to treat warts on the face since some treatments can cause scarring. Instead, contact a dermatologist. Also, seek professional help if the warts begin spreading.

•• **Appendix A** ••

A Parent's
Medicine Bag

A household with a child should be a household with a well-stocked medicine cabinet. The following list includes conventional medical supplies, nutrition supplements, herbal treatments, and homeopathic remedies that will probably prove useful in the treatment of common childhood illnesses and accidents. Additional remedies and products mentioned in the book are typically used less frequently and should be purchased as needed. All products should be stored out of reach of children, of course.

Conventional Supplies to Keep on Hand

- Adhesive tape: To secure gauze pads to the skin.
- Antiseptic cream: To kill germs and prevent infection caused by minor cuts and scrapes.
- Aspirator or bulb syringe: To remove nasal secretions in infants and toddlers.
- Calibrated dropper or spoon: To measure and dispense liquid medications.
- Decongestant: To relieve sinus congestion; use a children's formula.
- Humidifier: To add moisture to the air.
- Hydrogen peroxide: To rinse and disinfect minor cuts and scrapes.
- Painkiller: Acetaminophen, either in liquid, suspension

drops, or tablet form. Aspirin, including "baby aspirin," should never be given to children under age 18, due to the risk of developing Reye's syndrome, a potentially fatal disorder.

- Rehydration fluid: To provide water and electrolytes to children suffering from prolonged diarrhea and vomiting.
- Rubbing alcohol: To sterilize thermometers after use.
- Sterile bandages and gauze pads: To cover wounds and irritated skin after cleaning.
- Sunscreen lotion: To prevent sunburn in children 6 months old and older.
- Syrup of Ipecac: To induce vomiting in case of accidental poisoning.
- Thermometer (digital, oral, or rectal): To take the temperature.
- Tweezers: To remove splinters from the skin.

Nutritional Supplies to Keep on Hand

- Calcium
- Lactobacillus acidophilus
- Magnesium
- Multivitamin, multimineral daily supplements
- Vitamin C
- Vitamin E
- Zinc

Herbs to Keep on Hand

- Aloe vera
- Calendula ointment
- Chamomile tea
- Echinacea and goldenseal combination formula
- Garlic
- Ginger
- Licorice
- Oatmeal powder

- Peppermint tea
- Tea tree oil

Homeopathic Remedies to Keep on Hand

- Aconite
- Arnica
- Arsenium
- Belladonna
- Gelsemium
- Pulsatilla
- Rhus tox.
- Sulphur

•• Appendix B ••

Organizations
of Interest

Naturopathy

Naturopathic physicians are graduates of a 4-year postgraduate medical sciences program. Their training includes courses in herbal medicine, nutrition, homeopathy, exercise therapy, acupressure, and acupuncture. In 10 states—Alaska, Arizona, Connecticut, Florida, Hawaii, Montana, New Hampshire, Oregon, Utah, and Washington—naturopathic physicians (N.D.s) must pass a state licensing exam.

For a directory of qualified naturopathic physicians, contact the professional organization of licensed naturopathic physicians:

The American Association of Naturopathic Physicians
2366 East Lake Avenue East, Suite 322
Seattle, WA 98102
(206) 323-7610

There is a $5 fee for the information packet and national directory.

Holistic Medicine

Holistic Medicine is practiced by medical doctors (M.D.s), osteopaths (D.O.s), and naturopaths (N.D.s). These physicians emphasize the treatment of the whole person and encourage personal responsibility for health.

For a national directory of licensed holistic practioners, contact:

The American Holistic Medical Association
4101 Lake Boone Trail #201
Raleigh, NC 26707
(919) 787-5146

There is an $8 fee for the information packet and national directory. The Association also publishes the magazine *Holistic Medicine* 4 times a year; cost: $30 a year.

The American Holistic Health Association
P.O. Box 17400
Anaheim, CA 92817-7400
(714) 779-6152

Referrals and information are free.

Herbal Medicine

Herbal medicine is used by many naturopathic physicians and acupuncturists. There is no separate certification or licensing process specifically for practitioners of herbal medicine. Look for a practitioner who is a member of a professional organization, such as the American Herbalist Guild.

For information on herbal medicine and referrals to practitioners in your area, contact:

The American Herbalists Guild
P.O. Box 1683
Soquel, CA 95073
(408) 464-2441

Additional publications, newsletters, and books on herbal medicine are available from:

The American Botanical Council
P.O. Box 201660
Austin, TX 78720
(512) 331-8868
(800) 373-7105

Herb Research Foundation
1007 Pearl Street, Suite 200
Boulder, Co 80302
(303) 449-2265

Manufacturers of herb mail-order catalogs include:

East Earth Trade Winds
P.O. Box 493151
Redding, CA 96049-3151
(800) 258-6878
(916) 241-6878 in California

Herb-Pharm
P.O. Box 116
William, OR 97544
(503) 846-6262

Meridian Traditional Herbal Products
44 Linden Street
Brookline, MA 02146
(800) 356-6003
(617) 739-2636 in Massachusetts

McZand Herbal Inc.
P.O. Box 5312
Santa Monica, CA 90409
(310) 822-0500

Nature's Way Products, Inc.
10 Mountain Springs Parkway
Springville, UT 84663
(801) 489-1520

Windriver Herbs
P.O. Box 3876
Jackson, WY 83001
(800) 903-HERB

Acupressure

Acupuncture and acupressure professionals must meet state licensing or certification requirements in a number of states, including: Alaska, California, Colorado, Florida, Hawaii, Iowa, Maine, Montana, Massachusetts, Nevada, New Jersey, New Mexico, North Carolina, Oregon, Rhode Island, Texas, Utah, Vermont, Virginia, Washington, Wisconsin, and the District of Columbia.

For additional information on acupuncture and acupressure, as well as free referrals to several practioners in your area, contact:

**The American Association for Acupuncture and
    Oriental Medicine**
433 Front Street
Catasauqoa, PA 18032-2506
(610) 433-2448

Acupressure Institute
1533 Shattuck Avenue
Berkeley, CA 94709
(800) 442-2232
(415) 845-1059 in California

The Institute publishes a catalog of publications, videos, and products involving acupressure and Shiatsu therapy.

To confirm certification of a particular acupuncturist or acupressure practioner, contact:

**The National Commission for the Certification of
        Acupuncturists**
P.O. Box 97075
Washington, DC 20090
(202) 232-1404

Homeopathy

Homeopathy is practiced by medical doctors (M.D.s), osteopaths (D.O.s), naturopaths (N.D.s), chiropractors (D.C.s), and dentists (D.D.S.s). Some states also allow chiropractors, family nurse practioners, acupuncturists, and physician assistants to obtain licensure.

For an information packet on homeopathy and a directory of practioners, contact:

The National Center for Homeopathy
801 N. Fairfax Street, Suite 306
Alexandria, VA 22314
(703) 548-7790

There is a $6 fee for the information packet and directory. The Center also publishes the monthly magazine *Homeopathy Today*; cost: $40 a year.

The International Foundation for Homeopathy
2366 Eastlake Avenue E, Suite 301
Seattle, WA 98102-3366
(206) 324-8230

There is a $4 fee for the information packet and directory.

Manufacturers of homeopathic medicines that offer mail-order catalogs:

The Apothecary
5415 Cedar Lane
Bethesda, MD 20814
(301) 530-0800

Apthorp Pharmacy
2201 Broadway at 78th Street
New York, NY 10024
(800) 775-3582
(212) 877-3480

Bailey's Pharmacy
175 Harvard Ave.
Allston, MA 02134
(800) 239-6206
(617) 782-7202

Budget Pharmacy
3001 N.W. 7th Street
Miami, FL 33125
(800) 221-9772

Boericke and Tafel, Inc.
2381 Circadian Way
Santa Rosa, CA 95407
(707) 571-8202

Dolisos America, Inc.
3014 Rigel Ave.
Las Vegas, NV 89102
(702) 871-7153

Five Elements Center
115 Route 46W
Building D, Suite 29
Mountain Lakes, NJ 07046
(201) 402-8510

Hahnemann Pharmacy
828 San Pablo Ave.
Albany, CA 94706
(510) 527-3003

Homeopathic Educational Services
2124 Kittredge St.
Berkeley, CA 94707
(510) 649-0294

Homeopathy Overnight
4111 Simon Road
Youngstown, OH 44512
(800) ARNICA-30

Humphreys Pharmacal Co.
63 Meadow Rd.
Rutherford, NJ 07070
(201) 933-7744

Luyties Pharmacal Co.
4200 Laclede Ave.
St. Louis, MO 63108
(800) 325-8080

Santa Monica Homeopathic Co.
629 Broadway
Santa Monica, CA 90401
(310) 395-1131

Standard Homeopathy Co.
P.O. Box 61067
154 W. 131st Street
Los Angeles, CA 90061
(213) 321-4284

Taylor's Pharmacy
230 North Park Ave.
Winter Park, FL 32789
(407) 644-1025

Washington Homeopathic Pharmacy
4914 Del Ray Ave.
Bethesda, MD 20814
(301) 656-1695

Weleda Pharmacy, Inc.
175 North Route 9W
Congers, NY 10920
(914) 268-8572

Diet and Nutrition

For information on finding a qualified nutrition counselor, contact:

The Consumer Nutrition Hotline
(sponsored by The American Dietetic Association)
(800) 366-1655

The Hotline staff can answer questions and provide free referrals to registered dieticians in your area.

You can also request referrals to certified nutritional consultants by contacting:

The American Association of Nutritional Consultants
880 Canarios Court, Suite 210
Chula Vista, CA 91910-7810
(619) 482-8533

Publications on nutrition are available for a fee from:

American Institute of Nutrition
9650 Rockville Pike, Suite L4500
Bethesda, MD 20814-3990
(301) 530-7050

American Council on Science and Health
1995 Broadway, 16th Floor
New York, NY 10023-5860
(212) 362-7044

·· Appendix C ··

Additional Reading

Acupressure for Everybody by Cathryn Bauer. (New York, NY: Henry Holt and Co., 1991)

Acupressure's Potent Points by Michael Reed Gach. (New York, NY: Bantam Books, 1990)

Acupuncture: How It Works, How It Cures by Peter Firebrace and Sandra Hill. (New Canaan, CT: Keats Publishing Inc., 1994)

American Medical Association Family Medical Guide by J.R.M. Kunz and A.J. Finkel. (New York, NY: Random House, 1987)

The Complete Book of Homeopathy by Michael Weiner. (Garden City Park, NY: Avery Publishing Group, 1989)

The Complete Guide to Vitamins, Minerals, Supplements, and Herbs by Winter H. Griffith. (Tucson, AZ: Fisher Books, 1988)

The Complete Home Health Advisor: A Guide to Combining Standard Medical Treatments with Wholistic Alternatives by Rita Elkins. (Pleasant Grove, UT: Woodland Health Books, 1994)

The Complete Homeopathy Handbook by Miranda Castro. (New York, NY: St. Martin's Press, 1990)

The Concise Herbal Encyclopedia by Donald Law. (New York, NY: St. Martin's Press, 1973)

The Doctors Book of Home Remedies for Children by The Editors of Prevention Magazine Health Books. (New York, NY: Bantam Books, 1994)

The Encyclopedia of Alternative Health Care by Kristin Gottschalk Olsen (New York, NY: Pocket Books, 1989)

Encyclopedia of Natural Medicine by Michael Murray, N.D., and Joseph Pizzorono, N.D. (Rocklin, CA: Prima Publishing, 1991)

Everybody's Guide to Homeopathic Medicines by S. Cummings and D. Ullman. (Los Angeles, CA: J.P. Tarcher, 1984)

The Family Guide to Homeopathy: Symptoms and Natural Solutions by Dr. Andrew Lockie. (New York, NY: Fireside, 1989)

Food—Your Miracle Medicine: How Food Can Prevent and Cure Over 100

Symptoms and Problems by Jean Carper. (New York, NY: Harper-Collins, 1993)

The Food Pharmacy by Jean Carper. (New York, NY: Bantam Books, 1988)

Growing and Using the Healing Herbs by Gaea and Shandor Weiss. (Emmaus, PA: Rodale Press, 1985)

Herbal Healing by Michael Hallowell. (Garden City Park, NY: Avery Publishing Group, 1994)

The Healing Herbs: The Ultimate Guide to the Curative Power of Nature's Medicines by Michael Castleman. (New York, NY: Bantam Books, 1991)

Homeopathic Medicine for Children and Infants by D. Ullman. (New York, NY: J.P. Tarcher, 1992)

The Honest Herbal by Varro Tyler, Ph.D. (Binghamton, NY: Pharmaceutical Products Press, 1993)

Infant Massage: A Handbook for Loving Parents by V.S. McClure. (New York, NY: Bantam Books, 1989)

The Natural Family Doctor by Dr. Andrew Stanway with Rich Grossman. (New York, NY: Fireside, 1987)

The Natural Health First-Aid Guide: The definitive handbook of natural remedies for treating minor emergencies by Mark Mayell and the Editors of Natural Health Magazine. (New York, NY: Pocket Books, 1994)

Natural Health, Natural Medicine by Andrew Weil. (Boston, MA: Houghton Mifflin, 1990)

Natural Medicine for Children by J. Scott. (New York, NY: Avon Books, 1990)

The Natural Pharmacy Product Guide by Richard Israel. (Garden City Park, NY: Avery Publishing Group, 1991)

Magic and Medicine of Plants edited by Inge N. Dobelis. (Pleasantville, N.Y.: Reader's Digest, 1986)

The Parent's Guide to Pediatric Drugs by R.M. Bindler, Y. Tso, and L.B. Howry. (New York, NY: Harper and Row, 1986)

Prescription for Nutritional Healing by James and Phyllis Balch. (Garden City Park, NY: Avery Publishing Group, 1990)

Reader's Digest Family Guide to Natural Medicine: How to Stay Healthy the Natural Way by The Reader's Digest Association, edited by Alma E. Guinness. (New York, NY: Reader's Digest, 1993)

Rodale's Illustrated Encyclopedia of Herbs edited by Claire Kowalchik and William H. Hylton. (Emmaus, PA: Rodale Press, 1987)

Smart Medicine for a Healthier Child: A Practical A-to-Z Reference to Natural and Conventional Treatments for Infants and Children by Janet Zand, LAc, OMD; Rachel Walton, RN; Bob Rountree, M.D. (Garden City Park, NY: Avery Publishing Group, 1994)

Your Healthy Child: A Guide to Natural Health Care for Children by Alice Likowski Duncan. (Los Angeles, CA: Jeremy P. Tarcher, Inc., 1991)